USE AND APPROVAL OF ANTIHYPERTENSIVE AGENTS AND SURROGATE ENDPOINTS FOR THE APPROVAL OF DRUGS AFFECTING ANTIARRHYTHMIC HEART FAILURE AND HYPOLIPIDEMIA

DEVELOPMENTS IN CARDIOVASCULAR MEDICINE

Reiber, J.H.C., Serruys, P.W., Slager, C.J.: Quantitative coronary and left ventricular cineangiography. ISBN 0-89838-760-4.
Fagard, R.H., Bekaert, I.E., eds.: Sports cardiology. ISBN 0-89838-782-5. DICM 52.
Reiber, J.H.C., Serruys, P.W., eds.: State of the art in quantitative coronary arteriography. ISBN 0-89838-804-X. DICM 53.
Roelandt, J., ed.: Color doppler flow imaging. ISBN 0-89838-806-6. DICM 54.
van de Wall, E.E., ed.: Noninvasive imaging of cardiac metabolism. ISBN 0-89838-812-0. DICM 55.
Liebman, J., Plonsey, R., Rudy, Y., eds.: Pediatric and fundamental electrocardiography. ISBN 0-89838-815-5. DICM 56.
Higler, H., Hombach, V., eds.: Invasive cardiovascular therapy. ISBN 0-89838-818-X. DICM 57.
Serruys, P.W., Meester, G.T., eds.: Coronary angioplasty: a controlled model for ischemia. ISBN 0-89838-819-8. DICM 58.
Tooke, J.E., Smaje, L.H., eds.: Clinical investigation of the microcirculation. ISBN 0-89838-833-3. DICM 59.
van Dam, Th., van Oosterom, A., eds.: Electrocardiographic body surface mapping. ISBN 0-89838-834-1. DICM 60.
Spencer, M.P., ed.: Ultrasonic diagnosis of cerebrovascular disease. ISBN 0-89838-836-8. DICM 61.
Legato, M.J., ed.: The stressed heart. ISBN 0-89838-849-X. DICM 62.
Safar, M.E., ed.: Arterial and venous systems in essential hypertension. ISBN 0-89838-857-0. DICM 63.
Roelandt, J., ed.: Digital techniques in echocardiography. ISBN 0-89838-861-9. DICM 64.
Dhalla, N.S., Singal, P.K., Beamish, R.E., eds.: Pathophysiology of heart disease. ISBN 0-89838-864-3. DICM 65.
Dhalla, N.S., Pierce, G.N., Beamish, R.E., eds.: Heart function and metabolism. ISBN 0-89838-865-1. DICM 66.
Dhalla, N.S., Innes, I.R., Beamish, R.E., eds.: Myocardial ischemia. ISBN 0-89838-866-X. DICM 67.
Beamish, R.E., Panagia, V., Dhalla, N.S., eds.: Pharmacological aspects of heart disease. ISBN 0-89838-867-8. DICM 68.
Ter Keurs, H.E.D.J., Tyberg, J.V., eds.: Mechanics of the circulation. ISBN 0-89838-870-8. DICM 69.
Sideman, S., Beyar, R., eds.: Activation metabolism and perfusion of the heart. ISBN 0-89838-871-6. DICM 70.
Aliot, E., Lazzara, R., eds.: Ventricular tachycardias. ISBN 0-89838-881-3. DICM 71.
Schneeweiss, A., Schettler, G.: Cardiovascular drug therapy in the elderly. ISBN 0-89838-883-X. DICM 72.
Chapman, J.V., Sgalambro, A., eds.: Basic concepts in doppler echocardiography. ISBN 0-89838-888-0. DICM 73.
Chien, S., Dormandy, J., Ernst, E., Matrai, A., eds.: Clinical hemorheology. ISBN 0-89838-807-4. DICM 74.
Morganroth, J., Moore, E. Neil, eds.: Congestive heart failure. ISBN 0-89838-955-0. DICM 75.
Heintzen, P.H., Bursch, J.H., eds.: Progress in digital angiocardiography. ISBN 0-89838-965-8.
Scheinman, M., ed.: Catheter ablation of cardiac arrhythmias. ISBN 0-89838-967-4. DICM 78.
Spaan, J.A.E., Bruschke, A.V.G., Gittenberger, A.C., eds.: Coronary circulation. ISBN 0-89838-978-X. DICM 79.
Bayes de Luna, A., ed.: Therapeutics in cardiology. ISBN 0-89838-981-X. DICM 81.
Visser, C., Kan, G., Meltzer, R., eds.: Echocardiography in coronary artery disease. ISBN 0-89838-979-8. DICM 80.
Singal, P.K., ed.: Oxygen radicals in the pathophysiology of heart disease. ISBN 0-89838-375-7. DICM 86.
Iwata, H., Lombardini, J.B., Segawa, T., eds.: Taurine and the heart. ISBN 0-89838-396-X. DICM 93.
Mirvis, D.M., ed.: Body surface electrocardiographic mapping. ISBN 0-89838-983-6. DICM 82.
Morganroth, J., Moore, E.N., eds.: Silent myocardial ischemia. ISBN 0-89838-380-3. DICM 88.

USE AND APPROVAL OF ANTIHYPERTENSIVE AGENTS AND SURROGATE ENDPOINTS FOR THE APPROVAL OF DRUGS AFFECTING ANTIARRHYTHMIC HEART FAILURE AND HYPOLIPIDEMIA

PROCEEDINGS OF THE TENTH ANNUAL SYMPOSIUM ON NEW DRUGS & DEVICES, OCTOBER 31 - NOVEMBER 1, 1989

Edited by

JOEL MORGANROTH
LIKOFF CARDIOVASCULAR INSTITUTE
OF HAHNEMANN MEDICAL COLLEGE AND HOSPITAL

and

E. NEIL MOORE
SCHOOL OF VETERINARY MEDICINE
UNIVERSITY OF PENNSYLVANIA

KLUWER ACADEMIC PUBLISHERS
BOSTON DORDRECHT LONDON

Distributors for North America:
Kluwer Academic Publishers
101 Philip Drive
Assinippi Park
Norwell, Massachusetts 02061 USA

Distributors for all other countries:
Kluwer Academic Publishers Group
Distribution Centre
Post Office Box 322
3300 AH Dordrecht, THE NETHERLANDS

Library of Congress Cataloging-in-Publication Data

Symposium on New Drugs and Devices (10th : 1989 : Philadelphia, Pa.)
Use and approval of antihypertensive agents and surrogate endpoints for the approval of drugs affecting antiarrhythmic failure and hypolipidemia : proceedings of the Tenth Annual Symposium on New Drugs and Devices, October 31—November 1, 1989 / edited by Joel Morganroth and E. Neil Moore.
p. cm. — (Developments in cardiovascular medicine : v. 112)
ISBN 0-7923-0756-9
1. Cardiovascular agents—Testing—Congresses. 2. Hypotensive agents—Testing—Congresses. 3. United States, Food and Drug Administration—Congresses. I. Morganroth, Joel. II. Moore, E. Neil. III. Title. IV. Series.
RM345.S94 1989
615'.71—dc20 90-4492
CIP

Printed in the United States of America.

CONTENTS

SYMPOSIUM ON NEW DRUGS AND DEVICES
OCTOBER 31 - NOVEMBER 1, 1989
FACULTY

William B. Abrams, MD
Executive Director
Merck Sharp & Dohme
Research Laboratories

John C. Alexander, MD
Senior Vice President,
E.R. Squibb & Sons

Michael J. Antonaccio PhD
Senior Vice President
Bristol Myers Co.

J. Thomas Bigger, MD
Professor of Med & Pharm.
Columbia University

Aram Chobanian, MD
Dean-Boston University
Medical Center

Jay N. Cohn, MD
Head-Cardiovascular Div.
Univ. of Minnesota

William Frishman, MD
Professor of Medicine
Albert Einstein Hospital

John D. Irvin, MD,PhD
Executive Director,
Merck Sharp & Dohme

Norman M. Kaplan, MD
Professor of Int. Med.
UT Southwestern-Dallas

Peter Kowey, MD
Dir. Arrhythmia Serv.
Medical College of PA

Robert I. Levy, MD
President,
Sandoz Research Inst.

Raymond J. Lipicky, MD
Dir., Cardio-Renal Div.
FOOD & DRUG ADMINISTRATION

Harold K. Marder, MD
Senior Director,
Wyeth-Ayerst Research

E. Neil Moore, DVM, PhD
Professor of Phys. in Med.
University of Pennsylvania

Joel Morganroth, MD
Dir., Ctr. CV Studies
The Graduate Health System

Milton Packer, MD
Professor of Medicine
Mt. Sinai Medical Ctr.

Thomas G. Pickering, MD
Professor of Medicine
The New York Hospital

L. Ross Pierce, MD
Supervisory Med. Officer
FOOD & DRUG ADMINISTRATION

Betram Pitt, MD
Chief-Cardiovascular Div.
University of Michigan

Thomas Rector, PhD
Senior Research Assoc.
University of Minnesota

Eve E. Slater, MD
Executive Director
Merck Sharp & Dohme

Robert Temple, MD
Dir., Office of Drug Eval.
FOOD & DRUG ADMINISTRATION

Gloria Troendle, MD
Deputy Director
FOOD & DRUG ADMINISTRATION

Michael Weber, MD
Professor of Medicine
Long Beach VAH

William B. White, MD
Assoc. Prof. of Medicine
University of Connecticut

Preface

The Symposium on New Drugs provides for an annual forum for academic investigators, research and development personnel from the pharmaceutical and related health care industries, and members of the Food and Drug Administration to discuss important clinical research issues. The Tenth Annual Symposium on New Drugs addressed the problem of whether it was still appropriate to approve antihypertensive agents soley on the endpoint of lowering cuff blood pressure.

The initial discussions at this Symposium related to the approaches and methods to studying antihypertensive agents. Dr. William Frishman provided a detailed list of the new approaches to the treatment of hypertension and pointed out the many new concepts that are currently active in the development of many new antihypertensive agents. Dr. William White detailed the growing importance of ambulatory blood pressure monitoring to define hypertension and to determine the change in blood pressure due to pharmacologically active agents. Dr. Jay Cohn pointed out the flaws in using cuff blood pressure and detailed the potential virtues of using vascular compliance to identify patients requiring treatment for hypertension. Dr. Thomas Pickering also discussed the potential value of evaluating changes in left ventricular hypertrophy a finding which identifies high risk patients who need to be included in clinical trials. Dr. Michael Weber detailed the issues and suggested refinements in the approaches to clinical trial designs for antihypertensive agents and Dr. Raymond Lipicky discussed the definition of dose-duration and the role of non-Mem and Peak/Through measurements in defining an antihypertensive drug effect.

The second part of the Symposium reviewed FDA requirements for the approvability of new antihypertensive agents. Dr. Aram Chobanian detailed what had been learned from previous antihypertensive studies and Dr. William Abrams defined the specific studies required in the elderly patient and pointed out differences based on sex and race. Dr. Norman Kaplan reviewed the validity of a change in blood pressure as the only endpoint for approvability concerning possible and potential endpoints for the future. Dr. Harold Marder discussed the important issue of how the chosen endpoint effects the cost and time to develop a new antihypertensive agent and Dr. Robert Temple provided the FDA's viewpoint.

The potential for surrogate endpoints to provide an acceptable means of efficiently defining the risk versus benefit ratio for approvability of new drugs was another focus for this year's Symposium. Dr. J. Thomas Bigger discussed surrogate endponts for mortality in the study of antiarrhythmic drugs and Dr. Milton Packer defined the surrogate endpoints that might indicate benefit to the patient in the use of drugs to treat heart failure a condition in which the diagnosis is often imprecise.

Finally, Dr. Robert Levy provided a comprehensive discussion of the relationship between cholesterol lowering and cardiovascular disease endpoints.

We believe that the positions presented in these various manuscripts as well as the principles illucidated during the indepth panel discussions will provide the reader with a current state-of-the-art understanding of the current issues as well as the potential future directions in the evaluation of these cardiovascular therapeutic classes.

Joel Morganroth, M.D.

E. Neil Moore, DVM, Ph.D.

I. APPROACHES AND METHODS TO STUDYING ANTIHYPERTENSIVE DRUGS

1

NEW CONCEPTS IN ANTIHYPERTENSIVE DRUG THERAPY

William H. Frishman M.D.
Director of the Clinical Pharmacology Unit and Chief of Medicine, The Hospital of the Albert Einstein College of Medicine; Professor of Medicine, The Albert Einstein College of Medicine, Bronx, New York

There are many effective drug treatments for the management of patients with systemic hypertension (1). However, an ideal antihypertensive drug, which is both efficacious and free of adverse reactions, has yet to be introduced. This chapter will focus on new antihypertensive drugs at early stages of development (Table 1). These new agents have a considerable therapeutic potential, and represent highly selective pharmacologic approaches for the prevention and treatment of hypertension.

Table 1: NEWER CONCEPTS IN ANTIHYPERTENSIVE DRUG THERAPY

I Renin-Angiotensin System
- A. Renin inhibitors
- B. AngiotensinII-Receptor Antagonists
- C. New angiotensin converting enzyme inhibitors with diuretic and beta-adrenergic blocking activity.

II Atrial Naturetic Factor
- A. Atrial Naturetic Peptide Modulators
- B. C-ANP Receptor Antagonists
- C. Endopeptidase Inhibitors

III Potassium Efflux Stimulators
- A. Pinacidil and Cromakalim

IV Serotonergic Receptor Antagonists

	A. $5HT_2$ Blockers (ketanserin, ritanserin)
V	Serotonergic Receptor Agonists
	A. $5HT_{1A}$ Receptor Agonists (urapadil)
VI	Dopamine Receptor Agonists
	A. DA_1 Receptor Agonists
	B. DA_2 Receptor Agonists
VII	Adenosine Receptor Agonists
	A. P_1-Purinergic Receptor Agonists
VIII	Cyclic Guanosine 3',5-Monophosphate Phosphodiesterase Inhibitors
	A. Endothelium-Derived Relaxing Factor

Specific Renin Inhibitors

The converting enzyme inhibitors have been effective in the treatment of many patients with systemic hypertension (2) and/or congestive heart failure (3). A question that clinicians could ask is why any effort is being made to seek an alternative to converting enzyme inhibitor therapy. It appears that the major reason for looking beyond converting enzyme is its lack of specificity (4).

Recent efforts have focused on the inhibition of the renin-angiotensin system at other sites (Table 2), namely renin. Renin is considered an attractive therapeutic target for a number of reasons: 1) renin is the rate-limiting step in angiotensin II (A-II) synthesis; 2) angiotensinogen is the only substrate for renin, thus, unlike converting enzyme inhibitors, bradykinin should not be elevated; 3) molecular modeling information is available for renin (5).

Table 2: SITES FOR INHIBITION OF THE RENIN-ANGIOTENSIN SYSTEM

Step in the Pathway	Drugs
Renin biosynthesis	None available
Renin secretion	Beta-adrenergic blockers
Renin inhibition	Antibodies

Angiotensin converting enzyme	Captopril, enalapril, lisinopril; others to be released
Angiotensin II Receptor	Saralasin, non-peptide blockers

Renin has two aspartic acid residues in the active site which are essential for its catalytic activity.

Renin inhibitors include poly- and monoclonal antirenin antibodies which are very potent, and have been studied in animals and in humans (4-6). One of the first natural inhibitors was pepstatin, a microbial peptide. Pepstatin is a weak renin inhibitor and interacts with other aspartic proteinases (7).

More potent substrate analogue inhibitors have been constructed by substituting various nonhydrolyzable residues for the scissile bond (the peptide bond renin cleaves in angiotensinogen) (4). The most potent of these agents are believed to act as transition state mimetics (5). That is, agents which resemble the natural substrate at the scissile bond after being bound to renin (5).

The renin inhibitors, when given intravenously, can lower blood pressure without causing tachycardia in high-renin normotensive monkeys (8). Subsequent studies have shown that the fall in plasma renin activity with these agents is often but not always associated with a parallel reduction in blood pressure (5). In addition, some studies have revealed that the maximal fall in blood pressure occurs at doses far in excess of those causing inhibition of plasma renin activity (9). The recovery of blood pressure to pre-treatment levels also occurs more rapidly than the recovery of plasma renin activity (5). These data suggest that renin inhibitors may exert a hypotensive action unrelated to renin.

Studies in humans have reported reductions in blood pressure in both normal volunteers and hypertensive subjects (10,11). At this time, there is no evidence to support any major clinical differences between renin and converting enzyme inhibitors. Oral bioavailability and duration of action also remain problems hampering the widespread use of these compounds.

Angiotensin II-Receptor Antagonists

Non-peptide A-II-receptor antagonists may be considered a new milestone in the development of drugs interfering with the renin-angiotensin system (12). A selective antagonist of the A-II receptor would be able to affect the renin-angiotensin system independently of the source of A-II, including those alternative synthetic pathways which circumvent renin and converting enzyme (12).

A-II-receptor antagonists have consisted primarily of A-II analogues with saralasin representing the prototype agent (5). It is not orally active. The non-peptide receptor antagonists, which are tetrasubstituted imidazole derivaties, will be available for oral use in clinical trials.

New Angiotensin Converting Enzyme (ACE) Inhibitors

ACE inhibitors having other properties are now available which may provide advantages over the drugs currently available. There are converting enzyme inhibitors which possess diuretic actions which include naturetic and kaluretic activities (13). Agents are also available with additional beta-adrenergic blocking activity, albeit with stronger ACE effects (14). It is thought that drugs combining beta-adrenergic blocking activity with ACE activity would result in reduced A-II, while blunting the compensatory increase in renin release and the the cardiac response to sympathetic stimulation.

Atrial Natriuretic Peptide (ANP) Modulators

Evidence gathered over the past several years indicates that alterations in atrial natriuretic factor secretion or responsiveness are likely to modulate the expression of hypertensive disorders (15). Atrial natriuretic factor also possesses many attractive properties which would make it potentially useful for the treatment of hypertension (15). The well-known diuretic, natriuretic, and vasodilatory actions are complimented by other effects such as inhibition of renin, aldosterone, and vasopressin release (5,15).

In normotensive humans, the parenteral administration of ANP causes a prompt diuresis and natriuresis, a fall in systolic blood pressure, and a decrease in pulmonary capillary wedge pressure (16).

ANP is a large molecule structure and is not orally active (5,16). Efforts to synthesize smaller molecular weight peptides or peptides which are metabolically stable have been unsuccessful to date (17).

Receptors for ANP have been identified primarily in the kidney, brain, blood vessels, adrenal gland and intestine. Two receptor subtypes have been identified and characterized: the B-ANP receptor accounts for the biological actions of ANP; and the C-ANP receptor appears to function in the clearance of ANP from the circulation (5,16-18). Peptides have been synthesized that can interfere with the C-ANP receptors (19,20). It is possible that orally active C-ANP receptor antagonists can be found which elevate ANP by preventing its plasma clearance (5).

In addition to the clearing of ANP by a receptor mechanism, ANP is also metabolized by circulating endopeptidases (5). One endopeptidase inhibitor has been revealed which can cause cardiovascular activity similar to those seen with plasma ANP (21).

Potassium Efflux Stimulators

Agents which enhance potassium conductance are potent vasodilators (5). Newer antihypertensive agents representing this class are pinacidil and cromakalim but minoxidil is also believed to act as a potassium efflux stimulator (22). The agents are potent inhibitors of vascular effects of norepinephrine and epinephrine (22-24).

In animal studies, these drugs reduce peripheral vascular resistance and are accompanied by increments in heart rate and cardiac output (22,25). The tachycardia is sensitive to beta-adrenergic blockade (22). Associated elevations in plasma renin and catecholamines occur (22).

Pinacidil and cromakalim are effective antihypertensive agents. They are not practical, however, as monotherapies because of fluid retention and/or reflex tachycardia (26-28). They most likely will need to be used with a diuretic and/or a beta-adrenoceptor antagonist.

Serotonergic Receptor Antagonists

Agents that interact with serotonergic receptors (5HT) are of interest because of the proven effects on vascular smooth muscle and the sympathetic nervous system (29).

Ketanserin is a potent $5HT_2$ antagonist which exhibits antihypertensive efficacy in humans (30). Ketanserin is not only a $5HT_2$ antagonist but also a potent $alpha_1$-adrenergic blocker. Recent studies have shown that selective $5HT_2$ antagonists (ritanserin) are virtually inactive as antihypertensives (31). Thus, the mechanism of ketanserin is probably related to inhibition of $alpha_1$-adrenergic receptors. Perhaps the mechanism might be a cooperative interaction of $5HT_2$ and $alpha_1$-adrenoceptors.

Dopamine Receptor Agonists

Dopamine receptor antagonists are classified into two subtypes (DA_1 and DA_2) (5). The DA_1 receptors are predominantly postjunctional and are found on vascular smooth muscle of a number of vascular beds (32). The DA_2 receptors are found on presynaptic sympathetic nerve terminals, and modulate catecholamine release (32).

Fenoldapam is a selective DA_1 receptor agonist without $beta_2$-adrenergic agonist properties, and quinpirole is a DA_2 receptor agonist.

Although both agents reduce blood pressure and total peripheral resistance, their mechanisms of action are different (33,34). Fenoldopam is a direct-acting vasodilator which can act in the absence of sympathetic tone. It also antagonizes pressor responses to norepinephrine and A-II. The fall in blood pressure with fenoldopam is associated with increases in heart rate and plasma renin activity (5).

Quinpirole behaves like an indirect-acting vasodilator. The fall in blood pressure observed with the drug is associated with bradycardia, a decrease in plasma renin activity, and is dependent on pre-existing sympathetic tone. Quinpirole does not affect pressor responses to exogenously administered pressor agents (5).

Adenosine Receptor Agonists

Adenosine and analogs of adenosine interact with specific receptors affecting the cardiovascular system (5). Adenosine can modulate smooth muscle contractile force through a direct vasorelaxant effect, and also an inhibitory effect on neurotransmitter release (35,36). Recent studies have revealed that the direct effect of adenosine on smooth muscle is mediated by the adenosine receptor (37) and that inhibition of neurogenic contraction by adenosine is mediated by the $adenosine_1$ receptor (36).

$Alpha_1$-selective agonists have been studied in hypertensive animal models (37-39). These agents lower blood pressure without causing tachycardia. The agents are more potent where plasma renin is elevated since they also inhibit renin release (5).

Cyclic Guanosine 3',5'-Monophosphate Phosphodiesterase (c-GMP) Inhibition

c-GMP is involved in regulation of vascular smooth muscle contraction (40). Naturally-occurring vasodilators such as ANP, and drugs such as nitroglycerin, are believed to cause vasodilation by elevating c-GMP (41-43). Recently, efforts have focused on elevation of c-GMP by inhibition of phosphodiesterase metabolic enzymes (5). Agents in this class can lower blood pressure with parenteral use in rats (5).

Conclusion

In this chapter, a series of new approaches to blood pressure reduction have been proposed. It is not known which of these concepts will be most attractive for blood pressure control in humans. However, there is still a great need to develop antihypertensive drugs which deal specifically with the pathophysiology of hypertension in the individual patient.

References

1. Cressman, M.D., Vlasses, P.H. Med. Clinics N. Amer. 72 (2): 373-397, 1988.
2. Rotmensch, H.H., Vlasses, P.H., Ferguson, R.K. Med. Clinics N. Amer. 72 (2): 399-425, 1988.
3. Borek, B., Charlap, S., Frishman, W.H. Med. Clinics N. Amer. 73 (2): 315-338, 1989.
4. Haber, E., Hui, K.Y. In: Hypertension: Pathophysiology, Diagnosis and Treatment (Eds J.H. Laragh, B.M. Brenner), Raven Press, New York, 1990, pp 2343-2350.
5. Taylor, D.G., Kaplan, H.R. In: New Therapeutic Strategies in Hypertension (Eds N.M. Kaplan, B.M. Brenner, J.H. Laragh), Raven Press, New York, 1989, pp 125-139.
6. Dzau, V.J. J. Cardiovasc. Pharmacol. A53-A57, 1985.
7. Umezawa, H., Aoyagi, T., Morishima, H., Matsuzaki, M., Hamada, M., Takeuchi, T. J. Antibiot. 23: 259-262, 1970.
8. Greenlee, W.J. Pharmac. Res. 4: 364-374, 1987.
9. Blaine, E.H., Schorn, T.W., Boger, J. Hypertension 6 (Suppl 1): I-111-I-118, 1984.
10. Webb, D.J., Manhem, P.J.O., Ball, S.G., Inglis, G., Leckie, B.J., Lever, A.F., Morton, J.J., Robertson, J. I.S., Murray, G.D., Menard, J., Hallett, A., Jones, D. M., Szelke, M. J. Hypertens. 3: 653-658, 1985.
11. Zusman, R.M., Burton, J., Christensen, D., Dodds, A., Haber, E. Trans. Assoc. Am. Physicians 96: 365-374,

1983.
12. Timmermans, P.B.M., Carini, D.J., Chiu, A.T., et al. In: Hypertension: Pathophysiology, Diagnosis and Treatment (Eds J.H. Laragh, B.M. Brenner), Raven Press, New York, 1990, pp 2351-2360.
13. DeForrest, J.M., Waldron, T.L., Powell, J.R., Floyd, D.M., Sundeen, J.E. J. Cardiovasc. Pharmacol. 9: 154-159, 1987.
14. Allan, G., Cambridge, D., Hardy, G.W., Follenfant, M.J. Br. J. Pharmac. 90: 609-615, 1987.
15. Atlas, S.A., Laragh, J.H. In: Hypertension: Pathophysiology, Diagnosis and Treatment (Eds J.H. Laragh, B.M. Brenner), Raven Press, New York, 1990, pp 861-883.
16. Cody, R.J., Atlas, S.A., Laragh, J.H., Kubo, S.H., Covit, A.B., Ryman, K.S., Shaknovitch, A., Pondolfino, K., Clark, M., Camargo, M.J.F., Scarborough, R.M., Lewicki, J.A. J. Clin. Invest. 78: 1362, 1986.
17. Garcia, R., Thibault, G., Seidah, N.G., Lazure, C., Cantin, M., Genest, J., Chretien, M. Biochem. Biophys. Res. Comm. 126: 178-184, 1985.
18. Maack, T., Suzuki, M., Almeida, F.A., Nusenzveig, D., Scarborough, R.M., McEnroe, G.A., Lewicki, J.A. Science 238: 675-678, 1987.
19. Koepke, J., Tyler, L., Trapani, A., Bovy, P., Speak, K., Olins, G., Blaine, E. FASEB J. 2: A527, 1988.
20. Scarborough, R.M., Schenk, D.B., McEnroe, G.A., Arfsten, A., Kang, L.L., Schwartz, K., Lewicki, J.A. J. Biol. Chem. 261: 12960-12964, 1986.
21. Seymour, A.A., Delaney, N.G., Swerdel, J.N., Fennel, S.A., Neubeck, R., Druckman, S.P., Cushman, D.W., DeForrest, J.M. FASEB J. 2: A936, 1988.
22. Cohen, M.L. Drug Dev. Res. 9: 249-258, 1986.
23. Buckingham, R.E. Br. J. Pharmacol. 93: 541-552, 1988.
24. Cowley, A.J., Wynne, R.D., Hampton, J.R. J. Hypertens. 2 (Suppl 3): 547-549, 1984.
25. Cook, N.S., Quast, U., Hof, R.P., Baumlin, Y., Pally, C. J. Cardiovasc. Pharmacol. 11: 90-99, 1988.
26. Byyny, R.L., Nies, A.S., LoVerde, M.E., Mitchell, W.D. Clin. Pharmacol. Ther. 42: 50-57, 1987.
27. Izzo, J.L., Licht, M.R., Smith, R.J., Larrabee, P.S., Radke, K.J., Kallay, M.C. Am. J. Cardiol. 60: 303-308, 1987.
28. Vandenburg, M.J., Woodward, S.M.A., Stewart-long, P., Tasker, T., Pilgrim, A.J., Dews, I.M., Fairhurst, G. J. Hypertens. 5 (Suppl 5): S193-195, 1987.
29. Okin, S., Huberfeld, S.I., Frishman, W.H., Soberman, J., Laifer, L., Greenberg S., Lapsker, J., Charlap, S., Strom, J.A. J. Clin. Pharmacol. 28: 1008-1016, 1988.
30. Frishman, W.H., Okin, S., Huberfeld, S. Med. Clinics N. Amer. 72(2): 501-522, 1988.
31. Hosie, J., Stott, D.J., Robertson, J.I.S., Ball, S.G. J. Cardiovasc. Pharmacol. 10 (Suppl 3): S86-S88, 1987.
32. Hilditch, A., Drew, G.M. Clin. & Exper. Hyper. A9(5-6): 853-872, 1987.
33. Cavero, I., Thiry, C., Pratz, J., Lawson, K. Clin. &

Exper. Hyper A9(5-6): 931-952, 1987.
34. Hieble, J.P., Owen, D.A.A., Harvey, C.A., Blumberg, A.L., Valocik, R.E., DeMarinis, R.M. Clin. & Exper. Hyper. A9(5-6): 889-912, 1987.
35. Allgaier, C., Hertting, G., Kugelgen, O.U. Br. J. Pharmacol. 90: 403-412, 1987.
36. Paton, D.M. J. Auton. Pharmacol. 1: 287-290, 1981.
37. Herlihy, J.T., Bockman, E.L., Berne, R.M., Rubio, R. Am. J. Physiol. 230(5): 1239-1243, 1976.
38. Ryan, M.J., Mertz, T., Potoczak, R., Taylor, D., Kaplan, H.R. FASEB J. 2: A606, 1988.
39. Taylor, D.G., Bruns, F., Bjork, F., Cohen, D., Singer, R., Olszewski, B.J., Ryan, M.J., Trivedi, B., Kaplan, H.R. FASEB J. 2: A606, 1988.
40. Murad, F. J. Clin. Invest. 78: 1-5, 1986.
41. Rapoport, R.M., Waldman, S.A., Ginsburg, R., Molina, C.R., Murad, F. J. Cardiovasc. Pharmacol. 10: 82-89, 1987.
42. Takayanagi, R., Imada, T., Grammer, R.T., Misono, K.S., Naruse, M., Inagami, R. J. Hypertens. 4 (Suppl 3): S303-S-307, 1986.
43. Martin, W., Furchgott, R.F., Villani, G.M., Jothianandan, D. J. Pharmacol. Exp. Ther. 237: 539-547, 1986.

2

IS AMBULATORY BLOOD PRESSURE MONITORING REQUIRED TO DEFINE THE HYPERTENSIVE PATIENT AND TO DETECT EFFICACY?

WILLIAM B. WHITE, M.D.
Section of Hypertension and Vascular Diseases, Department of Medicine, University of Connecticut School of Medicine, Farmington, Connecticut, 06032

Introduction

Ambulatory monitoring of the blood pressure (BP) is a noninvasive clinical tool used in conjunction with mercury column sphygmomanometry that enables BP measurements outside of the medical care environment. During the past 20 years, automatic portable recorders have been developed which have greatly aided in assessing blood pressure during the day and night (1-3). There are a number of advantages of automatic ambulatory blood pressure monitoring (ABPM) over casual (or office) measurements in clinical hypertension research. The basis for the use of ABPM in place of or addition to the conventional clinic blood pressure (casual BP) is that numerous measurements over the day and night are more representative of both the directly-measured BP of an individual and the indexes of target organ damage associated with hypertension (4-6).

In addition to the important findings from a variety of cross-sectional studies that ABPM yields values that more closely predict pathophysiology than casual BP, ABPM introduces less observor bias into clinical trials (7) and is informative for both efficacy and duration of efficacy of the drug under question (4,8). Accordingly, this discussion focuses on the usefulness of ABPM in developing entry criteria for clinical hypertension studies and defining responses to antihypertensive therapy.

Evidence for ABPM having superior predictability of target organ disease in patients with hypertension

The basis for the pharmacologic treatment of hypertension is the excessive vascular damage, cardiovascular morbidity, and mortality seen in individuals with this disease. Thus, it has been necessary to demonstrate that ABPM is equal or superior to the casual BP in predicting the various indexes of cardiovascular morbidity or mortality prior to endorsing its use in clinical research or practice. A number of cross-sectional studies (5,6, 9-12) have now documented that ABPM is superior to the casual, clinic BP in predicting the presence of target organ involvement (retinopathy, impaired renal function, left ventricular hypertrophy) (Table 1).

Table 1. Studies Showing Superior Predictability of ABPM over Casual Blood Pressure for Indexes of Hypertensive Target Organ Damage in Mild/Moderate Hypertension

Author (ref)	*Target Organ Studied/Main Findings*
Asmar (12)	Peripheral vessels - ABPM superior in predicting distensibility/compliance
Devereux (9)	LV size by echocardiogram - Worksite BP predicts wall thickness better than casual BP
Opsahl (11)	Renal function - ABPM correlates better than casual BP for 24-hour albumin excretion
Parati (10)	LV size by ECG, retinal vessels - Intraarterial 24-hour BP and BP variability strong correlates with presence of target organ damage
White (5,6)	LV size (echocardiogram) and LV function (radioisotope) - previously untreated subjects - correlation only with ABPM and BP load*

LV - left ventricular ; ECG -electrocardiogram
** - Load defined as percentage elevated daytime (> 140/90 mmHg) and nighttime (> 120/80 mm Hg) BP*

There are a few studies to date (13,14) which have evaluated the prognostic implications of ABPM in patients with hypertension. The best known study has been that of Perloff and co-workers (13). They used a device known as the Portometer for measuring daytime ambulatory BP noninvasively and compared these data to clinic BP in predicting cardiovascular outcome following 5 years. The main finding was that patients whose daytime ambulatory BP was greater than their clinic BP had a greater rate of the cardiovascular complications of hypertension than individuals whose daytime ambulatory BP was less than the clinic BP. There are presently studies in progress which will further address the prognostic significance of ABPM, however, long-term 'natural' studies of hypertension are no longer considered ethical. Thus, it is unlikely that results from a large, prospective controlled trial of morbidity and mortality in hypertension using ABPM will be available.

Should there be new values of normalcy or abnormalcy for ambulatory blood pressure?

The generally accepted dividing line for normal versus abnormal BP has been 140/90 mm Hg for over 25 years. The use of this value has been strengthened by long-term natural outcome studies as well as by a variety of cooperative or multicenter antihypertensive drug trials. It is highly unlikely that the type of research that has brought us to the generally accepted values of borderline, mild, moderate, and severe hypertension via clinic or doctor's office measurements (15) will be replicated through similar ABPM trials.

In order to be practical, it has been our approach to utilize the generally accepted 'cut-off' values of the past 3 decades and apply them to ABPM rather than to attempt to develop new values. The one situation where a problem persists however, is in a cut-off value for BP during sleep. We recently have analyzed data from normotensive and hypertensive subjects that have undergone ambulatory monitoring of the BP and had both excellent records and no difficulties with sleep while wearing the recorder (4). In these populations, there seemed to be a natural 'cut-off' point of 120/80 mm Hg during sleep as the normal vs abnormal sleep BP in mild-to-moderate essential hypertensives (Table 2).

Table 2. Average Ambulatory Blood Pressure Values in Normotensive and Hypertensive Subjects

Parameter	Normotensives	Hypertensives
Office BP, mm Hg	**120/79 ± 9/6**	**151/101 ± 10/6**
24-Hour BP, mm Hg	**113/72 ± 9/5**	**139/87 ± 12/8**
Awake BP, mm Hg	**118/76 ± 9/5**	**149/93 ± 12/9**
Sleep BP, mm Hg	**98/60 ± 9/5**	**117/77 ± 9/7**
% Elevated Systolic BP*		
Awake (mean and range)	**11 ± 2 (0-33)**	**65 ± 7 (20-100)**
Sleep	**5 ± 2 (0-18)**	**52 ± 4 (10-75)**
% Elevated Diastolic BP**		
Awake	**10 ± 2 (0-18)**	**52 ± 4 (10-75)**
Sleep	**2 ± 1 (0-8)**	**53 ± 6 (5-100)**

(adapted from White WB, Morganroth J. Usefulness of ambulatory monitoring of the blood pressure in assessing antihypertensive therapy. Am J Cardiol 1989; 63: 94-98.)
*** - > 140 mm Hg while awake and > 120 mm Hg while asleep.**
**** - > 90 mm Hg while awake and > 80 mm Hg while asleep**

These 'cut-off' values of 120/80 mm Hg for sleep and 140/90 mm Hg while awake were tested in another study (6) to assess the ability to predict various indexes of cardiac involvement in hypertension. The correlations between percentages of abnormal BP while awake, during sleep, and during the entire 24-hour period (descriptively entitled the BP load) and the various cardiac indexes were compared to correlations obtained with casual and average ambulatory BP values. In almost every instance, the BP load was a stronger predictor of the cardiac indexes (left atrial size, left ventricular wall thicknesses, left ventricular diastolic function), than the mean ambulatory BP. Thus, the daily BP load can be used in lieu of average ambulatory BP values to predict the degree of target organ involvement in hypertension. This method of assessing ABPM findings not only simplifies data analysis but it helps to negate the need to find a 'new cut-off' value for average 24-hour, awake, or sleep BP. As will be discussed later, using the 'BP load' might also prove useful in assessing response to drug therapy.

17

Using Ambulatory Blood Pressure Monitoring to Form Inclusion or Exclusion Criteria for Antihypertensive Drug Trials

Numerous investigators have demonstrated the clinical utility of ABPM in assessing borderline and mild hypertension. A seminal finding resulting from the use of ABPM in clinical hypertension research has been the recognition of 'office' or 'white-coat' hypertension in as many as 12 to 20% of untreated mild hypertensives (16,17). Most investigators involved in ABPM methodology as part of an antihypertensive drug trial have recognized this phenomenon in patients who repeatedly will qualify for a mild or moderate hypertension study while on single-blind placebo therapy. Since these patients appear to be normotensive nearly all of the time that they are outside of the medical care environment (5,16,17) and they don't show target organ damage (5,6,9), it is unlikely that they will benefit from antihypertensive drug therapy.

Furthermore, there now have been a few reports evaluating the response that patients with 'office' or 'white-coat' hypertension demonstrate in clinical trials of antihypertensive drugs (18,19). These patients may appear unresponsive to therapy in the clinic setting (19). As their ambulatory BP values are generally normotensive on placebo, the out-of-office BP is nearly unaltered with active drug. In contrast, patients with hypertension both in- and out-of-the clinic (or office) demonstrate marked reductions in both clinic and ambulatory BP following drug therapy.

One might regard the 'office' hypertensives that enter antihypertensive trials as a *dilution factor* in the response to the agent under study. Thus, if ABPM is used in defining the hypertensive patient, the number of patients in the entire trial could be lessened since the power of the study will increase (8, 20). Utilizing both average ABPM values as well as daily BP load to define these individuals would enhance the specificity of the test and avoid placing individuals on drugs that probably offer little long-term benefit.

Use of Ambulatory Monitoring of the Blood Pressure to Assess Efficacy of Antihypertensive Agents

Present requirements. At the present time, ABPM is not required in the assessment of antihypertensive efficacy for a new drug application (NDA). What is presently required to demonstrate efficacy and duration of efficacy are short-term dose-ranging studies and longer-term safety and efficacy studies. The standard methodology used in antihypertensive studies is duplicate or triplicate supine or seated plus standing BP measurements in the clinic using mercury column sphygmomanometry (21). In 1987, incorporation of the so-called 'peak' and 'trough' measurements were added to dose-ranging and short-term efficacy studies. While not absolutely definitive (since every compound has its own characteristics), the *peak* pharmacodynamic response time of an antihypertensive compound is thought to occur when the hemodynamic effect of the drug is greatest (in contrast to the highest plasma concentration of the drug). The *trough* effect time of an antihypertensive agent is at the end of the dosing interval. General FDA guidelines state that the trough/peak ratio for ΔBP should be between .50-.66 to avoid both too little or too great an effect of the drug under study.

Practically speaking, obtaining peak and trough data is difficult in a wide variety of hypertensive subjects. It does require long periods of time at the research clinics or even an inpatient stay. Thus, demographics of the study group used for peak/trough calculations may differ from the general hypertensive population (e.g., only unemployed, elderly, retired may be able to participate in the study). Defining the peak effect of the drugs prior to the initiation of the study may be quite problematic. Often the peak effect is assessed in small groups of inpatients undergoing acute or very short-term dose-response studies. The observed peak effect in the phase II study may not be the same in the latter phase III study. Furthermore, it may not reflect what occurs in the ambulatory hypertensive patient. It has been our feeling that ABPM offers a more complete out-of-office assessment that can be applied to the general population (4,8).

Problems associated with ABPM. The methodology of ABPM is not problem-free. While the concept of its use is relatively simple, we have found that a variety of mechanical issues arise in multicenter drug studies (Table 3). Many of the prototype monitors were released for general use by their respective manufacturers without formal testing in the field. Thus, many of them were inaccurate, had software problems, or lost data from defects in the battery casing. Fortunately, the later versions of nearly all the monitors are much improved and accuracy and equipment failure are not really problems anymore (22).

Table 3. Technical or Mechanical Problems Associated with Ambulatory Blood Pressure Monitoring in Clinical Trials

- **Inaccurate equipment (applies mostly to older recorders)**
- **Lack of expertise of investigator and/or study coordinator**
- **Lack of interest of investigator and/or study coordinator**
- **Difficult patient populations: Obese, noncompliant, very light sleepers, patients with arrhythmias**
- **Excessive arm motion, soft K-sounds, loose ECG-leads (when applicable)**

Over the years, I have heard a variety of complaints from research directors at pharmaceutical companies with regard to multicenter ABPM studies. When the investigator or study coordinator at a particular site has not been scientifically or academically interested in ABPM, the technique is often performed poorly. Another problem encountered is the heterogeneity of patient populations at various institutions in a large trial. Obviously, certain individuals may be be less compliant with the recorder than others and excessive arm motion during the actual cuff deflation will inevitably cause technical problems (3, 22). However, I believe part of the problem with noncompliant patients is lack of patient education by investigators (or coordinators). Our success rate in Connecticut has been a direct result of discussing the mechanics and practical aspects of the recording with the patients in detail. When patients have a fairly good comprehension of the technique, they are more likely to keep their arms still, keep a good journal, participate for the full 24 hours, etc.

Data analysis for ABPM. There are a variety of ways to 'look' at data from an ambulatory BP study. The more commonly used techniques are listed in Table 4. None of these methods actually stand entirely alone in the assessment of efficacy or duration of efficacy. Statistical tests that apply to casual BP measurement often won't work out well with ABPM because of each individual's BP variability and the requirement to assess BP over time. Thus, it has been our approach to suggest the use of a combined method of assessment. To evaluate efficacy, the change in BP load will assess a statistical difference as well as evaluate response (e.g. control vs lack of control). Since the parameter of BP load has been validated as being well-related to the presence of disease (6) and helps to discriminate between borderline and mild hypertension (23), it should be one of the better means of assessing efficacy.

Table 4. Some Methods of Data Analysis with Ambulatory Blood Pressure Monitoring

- **Changes in 24-hour mean, awake, or sleep blood pressure on placebo versus study drug**
- **Visual appearance of 24-hour blood pressure profiles on placebo versus study drug**
- **Changes in BP over time (3- or 4-hour time blocks) in relationship to drug dosing**
- **Assessment of daily BP load on placebo versus study drug**

Assessing duration of efficacy with ABPM requires a large enough study group to take into account an individual's BP variability and unacceptable studies. Over a period of 24-hours, the standard deviation of the average BP is about 12-14/8-10 mm Hg. Most but not all patients have a marked reduction in BP during sleep and a large rise in BP soon after awakening. It is typical to dose patients early in the morning in these studies, place on the ABPM, and assess the next 24-hours after dosing. Unfortunately, the last 4-6 hour time block is usually when the patient is sleeping, has the lowest BP, and the least likely time to show an effect of the drug under study (24,25).

Thus, staggering the dosing time (and monitor placement) in the study population may be appropriate. If the drug was taken at noon for the purposes of the study, the time period between 0800 and 1200 the following day would be a representative 'awake' end of the dosing period for a once-daily agent. Since the BP (and hemodynamic parameters which contribute to BP) would ordinarily be elevated again, the effect of the antihypertensive drug may be more readily evaluable.

Sleep BP appears to have a significant independent relationship with indexes of target organ disease in hypertension (26, 27) and the lack of reduction of BP during sleep may exacerbate target organ disease (27). On the other hand, in most mildly hypertensive individuals with daytime employment, the BP during the times between 0200 and 0600 is generally the lowest of the 24-hour period. Thus, it may be that significant lowering of the BP during the middle of the night would result in excessive hypotension during the rest of the day and night.

Summary

Ambulatory blood pressure monitoring has evolved into a useful tool for assessment of pathophysiology and therapy in patients with hypertension. Accordingly, it has brought new insights into the heterogeneity of this disease and improves our diagnostic capabilities over the standard casual, office BP. These features, taken together with the abilities for BP recorders to assess drug effects over time, makes ABPM a superior methodology for defining the hypertensive patient and assessing efficacy.

References

1. White WB, Lund-Johansen P, McCabe EJ. Clinical evaluation of the Colin ABPM 630 at rest and during exercise: an ambulatory blood pressure monitor with gas-powered cuff inflation. *J Hypertension* 1989; 7: 477-483.

2. Harshfield G, Hwang C, Grim CE. A validation study of the Del Mar Avionics Pressurometer IV according to AAMI guidelines. *J Hypertension* 1988; 6: 913-918.

3. White WB, Lund-Johansen P, McCabe EJ, Omvik P. Clinical evaluation of the Accutracker II ambulatory blood pressure monitor: Comparison with sphygmomanometry, intraarterial blood pressure at rest and during exercise and assessment of performance in two countries. *J Hypertension* 1989; 8: in press (Dec).

4. White WB, Morganroth J. Usefulness of ambulatory monitoring of blood pressure in assessing antihypertensive therapy. *Am J Cardiol* 1989; 63: 94-98.

5. White WB, Schulman P, McCabe EJ, Dey HM. Average daily blood pressure not office blood pressure, determines cardiac function in patients with hypertension. *JAMA* 1989; 261: 873-877.

6. White WB, Dey HM, Schulman P. Assessment of the daily blood pressure load as a determinant of cardiac function in patients with mild-to-moderate hypertension. *Am Heart J* 1989; 118: 782-795.

7. Bruce NG, Shaper AG, Walker M, Wannamethee G. Observer bias in blood pressure studies. *J Hypertension* 1988; 6: 375-380.

8. White WB. Methods of blood pressure determination to assess antihypertensive agents: Are casual measurements enough? *Clin Pharmacol Ther* 1989; 45: 581-586.

9. Devereux RB, Pickering TG, Harshfield GA, et al. Left ventricular hypertrophy in patients with hypertension: Importance of blood pressure response to regularly recurring stress. *Circulation* 1983; 68: 470-476.

10. Parati G, Pomidossi G, Allini F, et al. Relationship of 24-hour blood pressure mean and variability to severity of target organ damage. *J Hypertension* 1987; 5: 93-98.

11. Opsahl JA, Abraham PA, Halstenson CE, et al. Correlation of office and ambulatory blood pressure measurements with urinary albumin and N-acetyl-beta-D-glucosaminidase excretions in essential hypertension. *Am J Hypertens* 1988; 1: 117S-120S.

12. Asmar RG, Brunel PC, Pannier BM, et al. Arterial distensibility and ambulatory blood pressure monitoring in essential hypertension. *Am J Cardiol* 1988; 61: 1066-1070.

13. Perloff D, Sokolow M, Cowan R. The prognostic value of ambulatory blood pressures. *JAMA* 1983; 249: 2792-2798.

14. Mann S, Millar-Craig MW, Raftery EB. Superiority of 24-hour measurement of blood pressure over clinic values in determining prognosis in hypertension. *Clin Exp Hypertens* 1985; A7: 279-281.

15. 1988 Joint National Committee. The 1988 report of the Joint National Committee on detection, evaluation, and treatment of high blood pressure. *Arch Int Med* 1988; 148: 1023-1038.

16. White WB. Assessment of patients with office hypertension by 24-hour noninvasive ambulatory blood pressure monitoring. *Arch Int Med* 1986; 146: 2196-2199.

17. Pickering TG, James GD, Boddie C, et al. How common is white coat hypertension? *JAMA* 1988; 259: 225-228.

18. Cheung DG, Gasster JL, Weber MA. Assessing duration of antihypertensive effects with whole-day blood pressure monitoring. *Arch Int Med* 1989; 149: 2021-2025.

19. Weber MA, Cheung DG, Graettinger WF, Lipson JL. Characterization of antihypertensive therapy by whole-day blood pressure monitoring. *JAMA* 1988; 259: 3281-3285.

20. Conway J, Johnston J, Coats A, Somers V, Sleight P. The use of ambulatory blood pressure monitoring to improve the accuracy and reduce the numbers of subjects in clinical trials of antihypertensive agents. *J Hypertension* 1988; 6: 111-116.

21. Fagan TC, Conrad KA, Mayshar PV, Mackie MJ, Hagaman RM. Single versus triplicate measurements of blood pressure and heart rate. *Hypertension* 1988; 11: 282-284.

22. White WB, Lund-Johansen P, Omvik P. Assessment of four ambulatory blood pressure monitors and measurements by clinicians versus intraarterial blood pressure at rest and during exercise. *Am J Cardiol* 1990; 65: in press (Jan.)

23. Zachariah PK, Sheps SG, Ilstrup DM, et al: Blood pressure load - a better determinant of hypertension. *Mayo Clin Proc* 1988; 63: 1085-1091.

24. White WB, McCabe EJ, Hager WD, Schulman P. The effects of the long-acting angiotensin-converting enzyme inhibitor, cilazapril, on casual, exercise, and ambulatory blood pressure. *Clin Pharmacol Ther* 1988; 44: 173-178.

25. White WB, Schulman P, McCabe EJ, Hager WD. Effects of chronic cetamolol therapy on resting, ambulatory, and exercise blood pressure and heart rate. *Clin Pharmacol Ther* 1986; 39: 664-668.

26. Murphy MB, Nelson K, Oliner C. Higher nocturnal blood pressure in normal and hypertensive blacks compared with whites. *Circulation* 1988; 78: II-569.

27. Smith VE, White WB, Karimeddini MK, McCabe EJ, Katz AM. Lowest not highest blood pressure predicts left ventricular filling. *Circulation* 1986; 74: II-73.

3

WHAT VASCULAR EFFECTS SHOULD BE MEASURED IN ANTIHYPERTENSIVE DRUG RESEARCH?

Jay N. Cohn, M.D.

Cardiovascular Division, Department of Medicine, University of Minnesota Medical School, Minneapolis, Minnesota

Although blood pressure measured by the cuff technique has served as the major criterion for the diagnosis of hypertension and a major endpoint for antihypertensive therapy, it is well recognized that this measurement is highly flawed:

1. Moment-to-moment fluctuations in blood pressure. Blood pressure variability makes any single measurement a poor reflection of the mean blood pressure over time. Indeed, this variability has led to a variety of responses including obtaining multiple readings at different times of the day, having the patient take his own blood pressure frequently throughout the day, and using intermittent recordings over a 24 or 48 hour period by an ambulatory technique. These techniques all provide additional data, but how these data are used in making a diagnosis or monitoring response to therapy remains controversial.

2. Inaccuracy of the cuff technique. Since the measurement of cuff blood pressure is an indirect assessment of intraarterial

pressure, a number of factors will influence the accuracy of the technique, including anatomical variations in the configurations of the upper arm, cuff width, bladder length, and tissue compressibility. Whereas systolic blood pressure by this technique may be quite reproducibly recorded by the appearance of the first Korotkoff sound, precision in the recording of diastolic blood pressure is difficult to achieve. The muffling and disappearance of the Korotkoff sound may occur at quite different pressures and there remains controversy as to which of these pressures should be recorded as the true diastolic pressure. Most studies suggest that the true diastolic exists somewhere between the muffling point and the disappearance point. Since the diastolic pressure is generally used as the major criterion for the diagnosis of hypertension, small changes in the recorded level may produce profound effects on diagnosis and treatment of the condition.

3. Systolic and diastolic readings are not an accurate reflection of mean pressure. The syndrome of hypertension is generally thought to indicate an increase in mean arterial pressure. Mean pressures are sometimes calculated from knowledge of the systolic peak and diastolic trough pressure, but in the absence of a full pulse wave which can be electronically meaned, this calculated mean may be significantly inaccurate. The contour of the arterial pulse wave may be so variable from individual to individual that the peak systolic pressures may provide

little insight into the mean systolic pressure and may seriously invalidate mean arterial pressures obtained from any standard formula.

4. Pressure correlates only weakly with cardiovascular events. Although in large populations there is an unquestionable relationship between systolic or diastolic arterial pressure and morbid cardiovascular events, this relationship is not very strong or consistent (1-6). Many hypertensive individuals go through life without any cardiovascular events, whereas most complications of ischemic heart disease occur in individuals without a prior history of hypertension. Therefore it is clear that the cardiovascular events that represent the major morbidity and mortality in the United States bear at best a weak relationship to the presence of hypertension and its severity.

These weaknesses of measured blood pressure as a guide to the diagnosis and treatment of hypertension have led us to search for a more specific marker. If we view hypertension as a vascular disease, then it would be appropriate to search for a vascular measurement which could identify the presence of the disease. Indeed, if the vascular abnormality is the prime defect in hypertension then elevated blood pressure might be viewed as an inconsistent manifestation of the disease rather than as the disease itself. The only vascular measurement which has been widely employed in the evaluation of the hypertensive patient is the calculated systemic vascular resistance. It is generally felt that a high vascular resistance is a hallmark of hypertension, but this resistance represents merely the ratio of mean arterial pressure to cardiac output and does not clearly discriminate hypertensive from normotensive individuals (7). The major site of resistance in the vascular bed is at the arteriolar level and a high resistance implies a reduction in caliber of the arterioles.

Arterial compliance is another vascular measurement which is a function not of the caliber of the vessel, but rather its distensibility in response to a pressure load (8). In the aorta and great vessels, the arterial compliance determines the storage capacity of the arterial bed during systole. In most prior studies in relatively normal young individuals, a figure of approximately 2 ml/mmHg has been obtained as the arterial vascular compliance (9). This value would indicate that at a pulse pressure of 40 mmHg as much as 80 ml of blood could be stored in the arterial vascular tree. Thus, the majority of the stroke time might well be accommodated in the arterial system during each beat. It is clear, therefore, that a reduction in arterial distensibility could have a profound effect on the characteristics of left ventricular ejection and on the arterial blood flow.

A second site of vascular distensibility is in the smaller arteries proximal to the arteriolar resistance vessels. These smaller arterial vessels will, if compliant, absorb some of the arterial pulse wave delivered to them and help transform the pulsatile wave form into the continuous wave form characteristic of capillary and venous flow. The pulse wave, however, also generates waves that reflect backward from these distal vascular sites providing a decaying sinusoidal wave that is superimposed on the arterial pulse wave generated from the left ventricle. This reflected wave may augment arterial pressure in systole and add pulsations to the diastolic pressure decay. The amplitude and frequency of this decaying sinusoid is very much dependent on the compliance of the distal arterial vasculature which serves as a reflecting point (10).

In order to gain insight into the vascular compliance abnormalities that may exist in hypertension, we have modified a technique originally described by Watt and Burrus utlizing pulse-contour analysis (10). This technique uses a computer algorithm to construct a third order equation, which can closely replicate the recorded diastolic pulse wave from the brachial artery in human subjects. By an independent recording of cardiac output, it is possible using this diastolic wave formula to solve the elements of a modified Windkessel model for the arterial vascular compliance (capacitive function) and the distal vascular distensibility (reflective function) (11).

In patients with hypertension studied in our laboratory, distal vascular compliance was strikingly reduced compared to age-matched normal subjects (12). The more proximal arterial compliance or capacitive function of the arterial circulation was only slightly and inconsistently lower in hypertensive individuals and appeared to be more intimately related to aging than to the presence of the vascular abnormality of hypertension.

The reduced vascular compliance in hypertension suggests that a decrease in distensibility of the vasculature in response to a pressure load may be a more sensitive and earlier marker for the vascular abnormality of hypertension than an actual elevation of blood pressure. Indeed it is possible that this abnormal stiffness of the vasculature is the physiologic marker for the hypertensive process. Furthermore, normalization of this reduced vascular compliance could be an appropriate therapeutic aim for pharmacologic management of hypertension. Only preliminary data are available to date, but it already appears that some antihypertensive drugs may be more effective than others in normalizing the arterial vascular compliance in hypertensive subjects (13). Considerable data would need to be collected on a wide range of patients treated with differing antihypertensive drugs to determine whether the measurement of vascular compliance will serve as a useful predictive marker for a favorable long-term effect of antihypertensive therapy.

Although monitoring of vascular compliance as a guide to the hypertensive disease process is just in its infancy, it is an attractive first step in an effort to identify a vascular abnormality that might characterize the disease process more precisely and consistently than does blood pressure or calculated systemic vascular resistance. In our early studies, it appears that distal compliance is strikingly reduced in all patients with diastolic arterial pressures above 120 mm/mmHg, but the vascular compliance in the normotensive and borderline hypertensive group is quite variable (12). Some individuals in this population have vascular compliance measurements well into the normal range whereas in others vascular compliance is strikingly reduced. The variability of arterial compliance measurements in these patients is not solely an effect of age. Thus, a low distal vascular compliance may be a marker for the borderline hypertensive subject who has the vascular abnormality likely to result in long-term complications of the hypertensive disease.

A number of possible virtues of this measurement as a guide to diagnosis and therapy need to be explored. The potential benefits of this measurement include the following:

1. Vascular compliance may be more reproducible than blood pressure and thus provide a vascular measurement not influenced by the day-to-day environmental and chronobiological effects that may influence measured blood pressure.

2. A reduction of vascular compliance corrected for age in any given individual might serve as a marker for hypertensive

vascular disease that needs to be treated. Currently many individuals with normal vascular distensibility may be treated for hypertension because their blood pressure is occasionally elevated. Eliminating such individuals from treatment programs and, particularily, drug trial protocols might increase the sensitivity of drug studies for lowering blood pressure and having a favorable effect on the vascular complications of hypertension.

3. Identifying individuals with low vascular compliance but normal blood pressures might identify a population who have a vascular abnormality prone to develop vascular events without hypertension. Drug therapy aimed at normalizing vascular compliance might have a favorable long-term effect in such patients even in the absence of a blood pressure lowering effect. Such a hypothesis certainly needs testing and could have a profound effect on the selection of patients for treatment in years to come.

4. Reduced vascular compliance is an important factor in the impedance to left ventricular damage and might be an important determinant of left ventricular hypertrophy quite independent from the actual blood pressure measurements. Furthermore, it is possible that drugs which have been effective in reversing left ventricular hypertrophy might be those who have a more profound effect on vascular compliance than drugs which have been

ineffective in reversing left ventricular hypertrophy. Studies of the relationship between drug intervention, vascular compliance, and left ventricular hypertrophy must be carried out to answer this question.

Vascular compliance may be only one of the possible measurements that can be used to identify the vascular abnormality of hypertension. The pulse-coutour method described in this paper represents only one of a number of methods that might be employed to characterize the stiffness of the vasculature. It is clear, however, that if more precision is to be achieved in identifying patients who need treatment for hypertension and if we are to be more forward in our effort to identify patients who are at risk for the development of vascular complications, then blood pressure measurements alone cannot serve as the sole guide to the diagnosis and treatment of this vascular process.

References

1. Medical Research Council Working Party. MRC trial of treatment of mild hypertension. Br Med J 1985;291:97-104.

2. Helgeland A. Treatment of mild hypertension: A 5 year controlled drug trial, The Oslo Study. Am J Med 1980;69:725-32.

3. Hodge JV, Smirk FH. The effect of drug treatment of hypertension on the distribution of deaths from various causes. Am Heart J 1967;73:441-52.

4. Chobanian A. Overview: Hypertension and atherosclerosis. Am Heart J 1988;116:319-22.

5. Devereux RB, Savage DD, Sachs I, Laragh JH. Relation of hemodynamic load to left ventricular hypertrophy and performance in hypertension. Am J Cardiol 1983;51:171-6.

6. Leenen FHH. Left ventricular hypertrophy in hypertensive patients. Am J Med 1989;86(Suppl IB):63-5.

7. Messerli FH. The hetereogeneity of essential hypertension: Hemodynamic aspects. Am Heart J 1988;116(2 pt 2):590-3.

8. Gribbin B, Pickering TG, Sleight P. Arterial distensibility in normal and hypertensive man. Clin Sci 1979;56:423-7.

9. Finkelstein SM, Collins VR. Vascular hemodynamic impedance measurement. Prog Cardiovasc Dis 1982;24:401-18.

10. Watt TB, Burrus CS. Arterial pressure contour analysis for estimating human vascular properties. J App Physiol 1976;40:171-6.

11. Finkelstein SM, Cohn JN, Collins RV, Carlyle PF, Shelley W: Vascular hemodynamic impedance in congestive heart failure. Am J Cardiol 1985;55:423-427

12. McVeigh GE, Burns DE, Carlyle PF, Finkelstein SM, Cohn JN: Vascular compliance in essential hypertension. Circulation 1989;80:II594

13. Zobel LR, Finkelstein SM, Carlyle PF, Cohn JN: Pressure pulse contour analysis in determining the effect of vasodilator drugs on vascular hemodynamic impedance characteristics in dogs. Am Heart J 1980;100:81-88

4

IS IT NECESSARY TO DEMONSTRATE CHANGES IN LEFT VENTRICULAR HYPERTROPHY IN THE EVALUATION OF ANTIHYPERTENSIVE DRUGS?

THOMAS G. PICKERING, M.D., D. Phil, and RICHARD B. DEVEREUX, M.D.

Cardovascular Center, The New York Hospital-Cornell Medical Center, New York, NY 10021

The ideal requirement for any new antihypertensive drug is that it should be shown to lower cardiovascular morbidity as well as blood pressure. In practice, this is unlikely to be achieved. The large scale clinical studies of the benefits of treating hypertension have produced findings that are both confusing and disappointing (1). While there is general consensus that any effective antihypertensive drug is likely to lower the prevalence of strokes, conclusive evidence that they prevent heart attacks is lacking, although this may be true of beta blockers in some patients. The costs involved in organizing and conducting a clinical trial where cardiovascular morbidity is the end-point makes it highly improbable that the newer agents such as calcium antagonists or angiotensin converting enzyme (ACE) inhibitors will be tested in this way.

The alternatives to this ideal approach are either to rely simply on the demonstration of a reduction of blood pressure, or to show an effect on intermediate markers of disease. Of these, left ventricular hypertrophy (LVH) is undoubtedly the most suitable, because it is thought to reflect the integrated effects of blood pressure over time on target organs, and has also been shown to be a potent risk factor for cardiovascular morbidity in its own right. In this review we will consider the implications of evaluating the effects of antihypertensive drugs on the regression of LVH.

Measurement of LVH. One of the chief advantages of incorporating LVH as a marker of hypertension is that it can be measured quite accurately, and is relatively stable over time. For the majority of hypertensive patients, M-mode echocardiography provides an estimate of left ventricular mass which has been shown to correlate very closely with actual ventricular mass measured at autopsy (2). The standard error of M-mode echocardiographic measurements is around 30g, and for serial studies the 95% confidence limits indicate that a change of left ventricular mass of 10g can be detected in a study population of 34 subjects or more (3). While large scale studies have for economic reasons relied on ECG assessment of LVH, echocardiographic assessment is much more sensitive and specific, and the extra cost is more than offset by the extra yield (4). Sensitivity of the echocardiogram for LVH is 85% or higher, whereas that of the ECG is less than 9% in the most recent analysis of Framingham data (5).

LVH as an integrated measure of blood pressure. The measurement of blood pressure itself is very unreliable, both because of the inherent variability of blood pressure and because of its susceptibility to transient emotional influences occurring at the moment of measurement. LVH is not susceptible to these disturbances, and has been shown in several studies to correlate more closely with ambulatory than with clinic pressures (6). Thus, it can be regarded as an index of an individual's "true" blood pressure. At the same time, blood pressure is only one of a number of factors which influence the development of LVH in hypertensive patients. Of these, the volume of the left ventricle may be the most important: in hypertensive patients with similar levels of blood pressure LV mass has been found to be higher in those patients with higher cardiac outputs (7), and LV stroke volume has been found to be as important a stimulus to LVH as arterial pressure (8). Another important factor is blood viscosity, which we have found to be more closely related than blood pressure to LV mass (9). There are almost certainly other less well understood factors, such as the effects of catecholamines, angiotensin, and genetic influences.

LVH as a predictor of morbidity. LVH may be regarded as an adaptive process in hypertension, since it operates to normalize wall stress, but there is increasing evidence that it is associated with a significantly increased cardiovascular morbidity, as compared to patients with similar levels of blood pressure and no LVH. This was originally shown by our own group (10), in a prospective study of 140 patients with initially uncomplicated hypertension followed over 4 years. Twenty percent of these men had LVH by echocardiographic criteria (LV mass greater than $125g/m^2$), and they had a fourfold higher incidence of cardiovascular morbid events than the men without LVH. These differences were independent of age, clinic blood pressure, smoking, and cholesterol. Similar findings have been reported by the Framingham study in a prospective 4 year survey of 1151 elderly men and women (11). Increased LV mass was a powerful predictor of coronary heart disease events which was independent of age, blood pressure, smoking, and blood lipids. More recently, we have extended our observations to a 10-year follow-up of 250 men and women with initially uncomplicated essential hypertension. LV mass greater than $125g/m^2$ strongly predicted cardiovascular deaths, all-cause mortality, and non-fatal cardiovascular events including myocardial infarction ($p<0.005$ to $<10^{-6}$), and in multivariate analysis only LV mass and age (but not blood pressure, gender, smoking or cholesterol) were independent predictors of adverse outcomes (12).

Why does LVH carry a poor prognosis? The adverse prognosis associated with LVH in a hypertensive patient could have at least three explanations: first, it may be that LV mass is a better measure of blood pressure than blood pressure itself, for reasons given above; second, there might be specific pathological effects of LVH on the heart; and third, myocardial ischemia may itself be a direct stimulus to hypertrophy. These possibilities are not, of course, mutually exclusive. Which is more relevant could in principle be determined by examining the morbid events associated with LVH: if the first explanation is correct LVH should be a good predictor of stroke; if the second and/or third are correct it should predict cardiac events better. In practice this is difficult to resolve because cardiac events as a complication of hypertension are so much common than strokes.

There is considerable evidence that the hypertrophied heart is more susceptible to ischemic and arrhythmic events. As outlined by Marcus (13) and Strauer (14), the basic problem is that the heart may outgrow its blood supply. Both animal and clinical studies have shown that myocardial infarction is less well tolerated when there is LVH, and coronary vascular reserve is also diminished. There is also evidence that patients with LVH have more ventricular arrhythmias than those without (15). In our ten-year follow-up study (12) cardiovascular death occurred in a higher proportion of patients who experienced morbid events among those with LVH than without it (55% vs 5%, p<0.005).

Regression of LVH as a result of treatment. Numerous clinical studies have shown that echocardiographically documented LVH can regress during effective antihypertensive treatment with drugs (16) or nonpharmacological treatments such as weight reduction (17) and sodium restriction (18). We have reviewed the results of several studies using different classes of antihypertensive drugs elsewhere (16), and concluded that there is a loose correlation (r=0.45) between the degree of blood pressure reduction and the regression of LV mass. There does, however, appear to be a difference according to the type of medication used. While sympatholytic drugs, calcium antagonists, and ACE inhibitors have all been shown to promote regression of LVH, this does not appear to be the case with diuretics and vasodilators (16). With the latter drugs, the lack of regression proportional to blood pressure reduction has been attributed to LV enlargement resulting from an increased cardiac output.

Is regression of LVH associated with an improved prognosis? Given that the presence of LVH has been shown to be associated with an adverse prognosis, it seems logical to suppose that regression of LVH is a desirable goal of antihypertensive treatment. Unfortunately, however, there is at the present time no direct evidence to support this possibility. While changes in ECG-LVH were evaluated in both the HDFP and MRFIT trials (19,20), the numbers of patients with LVH at the start of the trials and the insensitivity of the ECG method meant that it has not so far been possible to determine the effect of LVH regression on prognosis. Recent data from Framingham (21) suggesting that regression of LVH is prognostically beneficial have not yet been reported in a form that makes it possible to determine if this effect is related to hypertension or its treatment. It is possible that trials currently in progress, such as the Veteran's Administration Cooperative Study of Monotherpay of Hypertension and the Treatment of Mild Hypertension Study (TOMHS) may help to resolve this question.

A few studies have examined the effects of LVH regression on ventricular performance (22-24). Such evaluations are complicated by the fact that some indices of LV function should improve simply as a result of a reduced blood pressure (afterload). One index which allows for changes in afterload is wall stress, which has been found either not to change or to decrease as a result of LVH regression. Studies of diastolic function have also been reported during LVH regression, but their interpretation is even more problematic (25-26).

Conclusions. There is no doubt that evaluation of the effects of antihypertensive drugs on LV mass and function is a practical possibility, and that M-mode echocardiography is the method of choice. We have estimated previously that the high reliability of LV mass evaluation means that even with quite small sample sizes (e.g. of 15 patients) a reduction in mass of 7% can be detected. Furthermore, it is certainly of scientific interest to know whether any new drug does promote regression of LVH in addition to lowering blood pressure. The more important question for the present discussion is whether FDA approval of a new antihypertensive drug should be influenced by its ability or inability to promote regression. Here we enter the realm of speculation. The only class of drugs used as monotherapy which do not cause regression of LVH is the diuretics, and while there is considerable uncertainty as to their beneficial or adverse effects on coronary heart disease morbidity, there is no doubt that they are effective in preventing strokes. Therefore, while advocating the wider use of echocardiographic assessment of LV mass in clinical trials of antihypertensive drugs to resolve the question whether regression of LVH is associated with an improved prognosis, we believe that it is premature to make the demonstration of such regression a requirement for approval of a new drug.

REFERENCES

1. MacMahon SW, Cutler JA, Furberg CD, Payne GH. The effects of drug treatment for hypertension on morbidity and mortality from cardiovascular disease: A review of randomized controlled trials. Prog. Cardiovasc. Dis. 1986, 2(Suppl I) 99-118.
2. Devereux RB, Reichek N. Echocardiographic determination of left ventricular mass in man: anatomic validation of the method. Circulation 1977, 55:613-618.
3. Devereux RB. Detection of left ventricular hypertrophy by M-mode echocardiography anatomic validation, standardization, and comparison to other methods. Hypertension 1987, 9(Supp II):II-19-II-26.
4. Devereux RB, Casale PN, Wallerson DC, Kligfield P, Hammond IW, Liebson PR, Campo E, Alonso DR, Laragh JH. Cost-effectiveness of echocardiography and electrocardiography for detection of left ventricular hypertrophy in patients with systemic hypertension. Hypertension 1987, 9(Supp II):II-69-II-76.
5. Levy D, Labit SB, Anderson KM, Christiansen JC, Kannel WB, Castelli WP. Determinants of sensitivity and specificity of electrocardiographic criteria for left ventricular hypertrophy. Circulation (in press).
6. Devereux RB, Pickering TG. Relationship between ambulatory and exercise blood pressure and cardiac structure. Amer. Heart J. 1988, 116:1124-1133.
7. Hammond IW, Devereux RB, Alderman MH, Lutas EM, Spitzer MC, Crowley JS, Laragh JH. The prevalence and correlates of echocardiographic left ventricular hypertrophy among employed patients with uncomplicated hypertension. J. Am. Coll. Cardiol. 1986, 7:639-650.
8. Ganau A, Devereux RB, Pickering TG, Roman MJ, Schnall PL, Santucci S, Spitzer MC, Laragh JH. Relation of left venticular hemodynamic load and

contractile performance to left ventricular mass in hypertension. Circulation (in press).

9. Devereux RB, Drayer JIM, Chien S, Pickering TG, Letcher RL, Ye Young J, Sealey JE, Laragh JH. Whole blood viscosity as a determinant of cardiac hypertrophy in systemic hypertension. Am. J. Cardiol. 1984, 54:592-595.

10. Casale PN, Devereux RB, Milner M, Zullo G, Harshfield GA, Pickering TG, Laragh JH. Value of echocardiographic measurement of left ventricular mass in predicting cardiovascular morbid events in hypertensive men. Ann. Int. Med. 1986, 105, 173-178.

11. Levy D, Garrison RJ, Savage DD, Kannel WB, Castelli WP. Left ventricular mass and incidence of coronary heart disease in a elderly cohort. The Framingham Heart Study. Ann. Int. Med. 1989, 110, 101-107.

12. Koren MJ, Casale PN, Savage DD, Laragh JH, Devereux RB. Echocardiographically determined left ventricular mass predicts morbid events in hypertensive men and women--a ten year follow-up study. Clin. Res. 1989, 37:841A.

13. Marcus ML, Koyanagi S, Harrison DG, Doty DB, Hiratzka LF, Eastham CL. Abnormalities in the coronary circulation that occur as a consequence of cardiac hypertrophy. In: The Heart and Hypertension. Ed. FH. Messerli. Yorke. 1987, 231-240.

14. Strauer BE. Hypertensive Heart Disease. New York. Springer-Verlag. 1980.

15. Messerli FH. Clinical determinants and manifestations of left ventricular hypertrophy. In: The Heart and Hypertension. Ed. Messerli FH. Yorke. 1987, pp 219-227.

16. Devereux RB, Pickering TG, Cody RJ, Laragh JH. Relation of renin-angiotensin system activity to left ventricular hypertrophy and function in experimental and human hypertension. J. Clin. Hypertens. 1987, 3, 87-103.

17. MacMahon SW, Wilcken DEW, MacDonald GJ. The effect of weight reduction on left ventricular mass: A randomized controlled trial in young, overweight, hypertensive patients. N. Engl. J. Med. 1986, 314:334-339.

18. Ferrara LA, DeSimone G, Pasanisi F, Mancini M, Mancini M. Left ventricular mass reduction during salt depletion in arterial hypertension. Hypertension. 1984, 6, 755-759.

19. Hypertension Detection and Follow-up Program Cooperative Group. Five year findings of the Hypertension Detection and Follow-up Program. Prevention and reversal of left ventricular

hypertrophy with antihypertensive drug therapy. Hypertension. 1985, 7, 105-112.

20. MacMahon A, Collins G, Rautahaharju P, . Electro-cardiographic left ventricular hypertrophy and effects of anti-hypertensive drug therapy in hypertensive drug therapy in hypertensive participants in the Multiple Risk Factor Intervention Trial. Amer. J. Cardiol. 1989, 63, 202-210.
21. Kannel WB, D'Agostino RB, Levy D, Belanger AJ. Prognostic significance of regression of left ventricular hypertrophy. (Abstr) Circulation, 1988 (Suppl II): I-89.
22. Dunn FG, Ventura HO, Messerli FH, Kobrin I, Frohlich ED. Time course of regression of left ventricular hypertrophy in hypertensive patients treated with atenolol. Circulation 1987, 76, 254-258.
23. Nakashima Y, Fouad FM, Tarazi RC. Regression of left ventricular hypertrophy from systemic hypertension by enalapril. Am. J. Cardiol. 1984, 53, 1044-1049.
24. Liebson PR, Savage DD. Echocardiography in hypertension: A review II. Echocardiographic studies of the effects of antihypertensive agents on left ventricular wall mass and function. Echocardiogaphy 1987, 4, 215-249.
25. Szlachic J, Tubau JF, Vollmer C, Massie BM. Effects of diltiazem on left ventricular mass and diastolic filling in mild to moderate hypertension. Amer. J. Cardiol. 1989, 63, 198-201.
26. White WB, Schulman P, Karimeddin MK, Smith VE. Regression of left ventricular mass is accompanied by improvement in rapid left ventricular filling following antihypertensive therapy with atenolol. Amer. Heart J. 1989, 117,145-150.

5

CLINICAL TRIALS OF ANTIHYPERTENSIVE AGENTS

M. A. WEBER, J. M. NEUTEL, D. H. G. SMITH

Hypertension Center, Department of Medicine, VA Medical Center, Long Beach; University of California, Irvine, CA

ABSTRACT

Clinical trials of the efficacy of new antihypertensive agents have two principal aims: to define the effective dose range for each drug and to establish its duration of action. There is no ideal trial design for dose ranging. The conventionally used parallel groups design is probably the most practical and allows estimates of response rates at each dose level. Crossover or ascending dose studies may generate dose-response curves that are more relevant clinically, but they are of far longer duration. Recent studies with automated whole-day blood pressure monitoring have shown that standard assumptions about drug duration of action may be misleading. This paper examines these issues and makes suggestions for refining some of the present approaches. We have also briefly looked at practical questions, including problems associated with the diagnosis of hypertension, patients previously on antihypertensive therapy, entry criteria for protocols, and unexpected placebo effects.

INTRODUCTION

Hypertension is still a young discipline that until now has been characterized largely by epidemiologic methods. We still have much to learn about its causes, prognosis and the effects of treatment in the individual patient. Because research in hypertension is now in such a dynamic phase, it follows that the goals of therapeutic studies are continually changing.

Inevitably, the design of clinical trials of new antihypertensive agents, including protocols used for obtaining approval for marketing in the United States, must reflect these changes. The traditional assumption underlying therapy is that hypertension is a strong risk factor for such cardiovascular events as strokes, heart failure, myocardial infarction and renal insufficiency. Therefore, the rationale for treatment is that the incidence of these events in hypertensive patients can be reduced.

The Food and Drug Administration, however, has adopted the view that efficacy of antihypertensive agents is established when they can be shown to decrease blood pressure significantly when compared with placebo. No other end point of treatment need be demonstrated. This policy is justified by earlier large-scale clinical trials that reported decreases in vascular complications when patients where given blood pressure-lowering drugs. Moreover, the FDA acknowledges that these types of clinical end points would be excessively burdensome and expensive in the testing of new agents.

In evaluating efficacy, the FDA is interested in two primary issues: the appropriate range of doses for an agent, and its duration of effect. From these data, it should be possible to write a label that provides helpful information to the prescriber on the selection of appropriate doses and the frequency with which they should be administered. There has been controversy over the best trial designs for establishing dose ranges and dosing intervals, and these will be discussed in more detail below. It is also well established that many patients, perhaps a majority, require two or more drugs to control their hypertension. Studies of antihypertensive agents in combination is another issue that will be considered further.

One other matter also now appears important in studies of antihypertensive efficacy. It is apparent that although high blood pressure is an independent risk factor for cardiovascular events, it has a close link, perhaps on a genetic basis, with other factors that determine the likelihood of vascular episodes. Dyslipidemias, abnormalities of insulin and glucose metabolism, and hypertrophic vascular changes all appear to be important in this context. Documenting the effects of antihypertensive therapy on the broader range of risk factors now appears to be an essential part of clinical trials.

OPERATIONAL ISSUES IN ANTIHYPERTENSIVE TRIALS

The development of several new antihypertensive agents during the past few years has helped standardize methods for enrolling patients in protocols, allocating them to treatment, and observing the effects of drugs on efficacy and other clinical parameters. Apart from study design issues involved with the measurements of dose ranges and dosing intervals, there are questions about some of the methodology details in antihypertensive clinical trials.

Selection of Appropriate Patients.

Copious experience now dictates criteria for accepting patients into studies and rejecting those who are not suitable. There are some unavoidable blemishes in this process. Antihypertensive trials tend to exclude many patients with concurrent cardiovascular or other conditions, or who are taking concurrent medications for separate chronic conditions. These patients, in reality, are typical of those encountered in clinical practice. But there is a problem of a more technical nature: finding patients who are truly hypertensive, and whose pre-treatment blood pressures are at a constant level.

The Diagnosis Problem. Despite the care with which patients typically are evaluated prior to study entry, major hypertension trials have reported that between 20-40% of placebo-treated patients experience substantial blood pressure reductions by the end of study (1,2). It seems probable that the hypertension in the majority of these patients was initially misdiagnosed. Observations with automated whole-day ambulatory blood pressure monitoring techniques have confirmed that at least one-quarter of patients evaluated in the conventional clinical setting (3) or entering formal antihypertensive trials (4) have an erroneous diagnosis. There may be important differences between true hypertensives and misdiagnosed hypertensives in their responses to treatment. As practicing clinicians become more aware of this problem, it would be helpful for antihypertensive trials to become more rigorous in establishing the correct diagnosis. Indeed, the problem may already be worse in trial patients than in standard clinical practice, for investigators are often motivated into rapidly recruiting patients who are near the borderline of the blood pressure entry criteria.

The Shifting Baseline. Many patients entering antihypertensive trials have already been receiving therapy or have been participating in a previous trial. The usual routine is to subject such patients to a "washout period" during which their earlier treatment is discontinued and their blood pressures are allowed to rise back into the hypertensive range. There is growing evidence, however, that blood pressures in these patients are not allowed to return completely to their hypertensive baselines. Studies using ambulatory blood pressure monitoring during antihypertensive trials have shown that blood pressure values in placebo-treated patients actually may rise by 3-5 mmHg during a typical 6 to 8 week study period. The explanation for this phenomenon is not clear, but could reflect unexpectedly long durations of action of previous therapy. It is also possible that more fundamental mechanisms, including baroreceptor sensitivity, autoregulation responses, and peripheral arterial smooth muscle hypertrophy may require several weeks following treatment discontinuation to return to their true baseline status.

Suggestion. The washout periods may not be sufficiently long. A common practice, although not mandated by the FDA, is that patients completing one trial switch to a thirty day period of conventional treatment before entering the washout period of a new trial. It may be more appropriate for patients to remain completely free of treatment (provided that there are no unacceptable risks or other practical problems) between studies, allowing investigators to ensure that these patients have returned fully to their untreated status. Antihypertensive trials conventionally require entry blood pressure values during two consecutive visits that are within 5 to 7 mmHg of each other. This criterion may not be sufficiently rigorous: firstly, it is important to ensure that any differences between these readings do not indicate a continuing upward trend in the blood pressure; and secondly, ensuring a constancy of blood pressures during periods greater than just one week (provided that there are no safety concerns) should also minimize the problems of unreliable baselines.

Placebo Subtraction.

In studies based on the parallel groups design, effects observed within the placebo group are subtracted from the effects in the actively treated groups, thus providing a measurement of the true efficacy of the drug. But this approach might lead to inaccurate estimates in some patients, especially those with mild hypertension. To facilitate rapid patient entry into studies, investigators sometimes appear to inadvertently use an upward digit preference during the blood pressure measurements, thereby assisting patients to achieve entry criteria (typically a diastolic BP of 95 mmHg). Later in the study there is the possibility of a downward digit preference during BP measurement to help patients achieve goals of treatment response (typically a diastolic BP of 90 mmHg). Thus, exaggerated reductions in blood pressure might be created for placebo-treated patients enrolled near the low end of the blood pressure entry criteria. Indeed, analysis of recent data has shown that placebo antihypertensive effects appear to be greater in patients with entry diastolic blood pressures below 100 mmHg than in those with entry readings above 100 mmHg; this pattern is opposite to that found with active drug therapy, where treatment usually produces its greatest effects in patients with high entry blood pressures. Although the exaggerated placebo effect may be comparatively small (2 to 3 mmHg greater than the "true" effect), it may have an important impact when subtracted from the relatively modest active drug effects occurring at the end of dosing intervals.

Suggestion. A solution to this problem could be the wider use of the relatively blinded random zero sphygmomanometer; alternatively, reliable electronic blood pressure-measuring devices might provide the most truly objective readings.

Heterogeneity of Hypertension.

The nature of essential hypertension is still not well understood. Clearly, several separate mechanisms can contribute to this condition. For this reason, antihypertensive drugs have a lower efficacy rate than some other types of pharmacological agents. Clinically meaningful decreases in blood pressure occur in only 40-50% of hypertensive patients treated with single agents. This problem is readily dealt with in clinical practice where either a second drug is added or the unsuccessful agent is replaced.

Unfortunately, this logical approach cannot easily be built into large-scale clinical trials, and the effects in responding and nonresponding patients are averaged together. This is not really a relevant process. Instead, it might be more valid to express results in terms of response rates. This might be especially important when evaluating "trough" data at the end of dosing intervals, where it seems inappropriate to analyze duration of drug action in individuals in whom there has been no meaningful drug action. This problem will be considered below in the discussion on dosing frequency.

Evaluation of Risk Factors.

As discussed by other authors in this Volume, there are interrelationships between hypertension and other cardiovascular risk factors that appear to have a more powerful impact on clinical outcome than would be expected from consideration of the risk factors individually. Awareness of this problem should be reflected in study design. For example, epidemiologic data and therapeutic trials (5) have demonstrated a synergy between blood pressure and lipid abnormalities both in predicting coronary events and in determining the impact of treatment on these events. It is clear, too, that antihypertensive drugs have differential effects on insulin and glucose metabolism, again potentially a vital factor in determining outcome of treatment. The presence of left ventricular hypertrophy in hypertensive patients may be a more important predictor of cardiovascular events than blood pressure itself, again raising important therapeutic implications. Practicing clinicians have become sensitive to these issues, and are starting to decrease their use of such agents as diuretics which, despite their antihypertensive efficacy, may have adverse or unhelpful actions on other risk factors. It is not suggested that we stop using blood pressure effects themselves as the primary endpoints of antihypertensive trials. Nevertheless, studies of the actions of antihypertensive drugs on these differing risk factors should no longer be perceived simply as safety issues or as subjects for late phase marketing studies. Instead, they should be regarded as fundamental pharmacologic properties to be studied as part of characterizing new antihypertensive agents.

Automated Blood Pressure Monitoring.

Other authors in this Volume will describe in detail the use and application of whole-day ambulatory blood pressure monitoring techniques in the evaluation of antihypertensive agents. Yet, in this discussion of antihypertensive trial design, it is also necessary to indicate the importance of these new approaches. Automated blood pressure monitoring provides enhanced power for analysis, allowing conclusions to be reached with fewer patients than with conventional measurements. These techniques also provide clear data on duration of action of antihypertensive agents, and enable scrutiny of blood pressure effects at important times of day (including the early to mid-morning hours) that are not accessible to standard clinical observations. The accuracy, reliability and convenience of the portable devices have been improved substantially during the past few years, and it now appears appropriate to recommend their use on a routine basis for clinical trials of new antihypertensive agents.

THE DOSE RANGE

Establishing a dose range for new antihypertensive agents is one of the major priorities of the FDA guidelines. There is an assumption that these agents can describe a dose-response curve, and it is thus appropriate to define the lower and upper limits of the effective dose range. Specifically, the FDA asks that the minimum effective dose and the maximum dose (beyond which there is no further therapeutic effect) be defined. From the physician's point of view, four pieces of information are important: the reasonable starting dose; appropriate dose increments when blood pressures fail to respond adequately to the starting dose; the maximum dose that should be tried; and perhaps most important of all, the dose level most likely to be successful.

Surveys of the prescribing habits of clinicians indicate that they tend to be cautious in choosing doses, often leaving their patients on ineffective treatment at the low end of the dose range. Indeed, it is interesting that the FDA has approved the marketing of dosage strengths of antihypertensive agents (especially the ACE inhibitors and alpha blockers) that fall below the minimum dose levels required to produce meaningful clinical effects. Analysis of data should be orientated to provide physicians with response rates at different dose levels, thus providing a basis for realistic selection of drug strengths.

Duration and Amplitude of Effects.

There is much that we do not understand about the ways in which antihypertensive agents produce their effects. There is not a well established relationship between the pharmacokinetics of these drugs and their hemodynamic properties. With at least some drug classes, however, dose size correlates more closely with the duration of antihypertensive effect than with its amplitude. Thus, physicians who see their patients during their mid-morning office hours, typically just 2-3 hours after dosing, may be mislead into attributing efficacy to inappropriately low doses. From the study design point of view, obviously it is mandatory to study blood pressure effects at the end of the dosing intervals when constructing dose-response curves.

Implicit in this approach is the assumption that a reasonable dosing interval can be selected. For marketing reasons, there has been an understandable tendency by drug manufacturers to select relatively long intervals, frequently 24 hours. Unfortunately, efficacy with drugs administered once daily sometimes requires very high doses. A typical problem of this type is illustrated in Figure 1 (6), where the blood pressure reduction 24 hours after dosing is relatively modest despite the use of doses far higher than are usually prescribed.

Study Designs for Dose Ranging.

The current belief of the FDA is that doses are best defined by the use of so-called parallel groups studies. Other possible approaches advocated by clinical pharmacologists include crossover designs (of which the individual patient N of 1 design is an example), and dose escalation studies (also known as titration studies).

Parallel Groups Design.

In this study design patients are allocated randomly to receive either placebo or one of several differing doses of active drug throughout the study. Once allocated, patients do not change their treatment. From these data it is possible to construct a dose response curve starting with the placebo effect and comparing it with the differing doses of drug. A criticism of this approach (7) is that each patient participates at only one point of the dose response curve. It has been argued that the dose response curve achieved from the parallel groups design is not identical to the curve derived from the pooling of multiple dose response curves obtained from within individual patients (7). It is not clear whether the parallel groups approach to dose response curves provides data that are deficient in the clinical context. Advantages of the parallel groups approach are that the study design is simple and of relatively short duration. It can also provide information concerning the therapeutic response rate at each dose level.

Crossover Design.

This design also employs treatment with placebo and the differing doses of active drug, but each patient is exposed to each possible type of treatment. The sequence of treatments within each individual patient is randomized. This type of design has more statistical power than the parallel groups approach, and thus requires fewer patients. Moreover, it enables dose response curves to be developed for each individual participant. Unfortunately, this type of study is of considerable duration and expense unless it is restricted to placebo and just one or two drug dosage

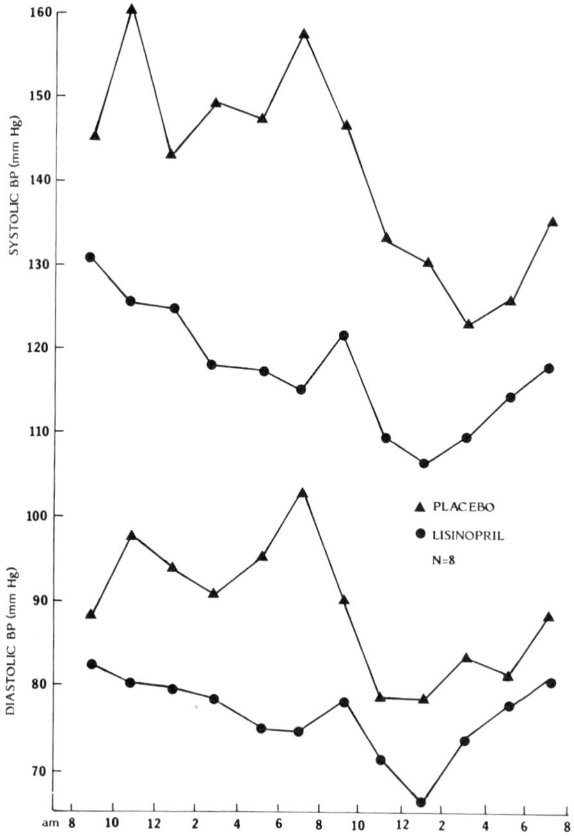

Fig. 1. Baseline (triangles) and treatment (circles) blood pressure values in patients treated with lisinopril monotherapy. Doses were titrated so as to achieve efficacy at trough (8:00 am), and ranged from 40 to 80 mg (mean:70 mg).

levels. Even then, if appropriate between-treatment washout periods are employed, the time commitment can be unacceptable. Crossover studies may be more appropriate for direct comparisons between antihypertensive agents, especially if single or highly simplified dosage regimens are employed. Crossover studies may also be valuable in studying the efficacy of antihypertensive drug combinations, and are considered later.

There has been some recent interest in the so-called N of 1 randomized controlled trial (8). This has been recommended as an approach for practicing clinicians to seek out an optimal treatment or drug dosage in individual patients. In essence, patients are exposed to a crossover design in which placebo treatment and differing drug doses are tested in a randomized sequence. Hypertension is a suitable condition for using this type of trial design. Its application to larger scale experiences that could lead to generalized recommendations to practitioners has yet to be established.

Dose Escalation Design.

This design, sometimes called titration studies, is similar to the crossover approach in that each patient potentially is exposed to placebo and each dosage level of active drug. The critical difference, however, is that the doses are administered in ascending fashion rather than in a randomized sequence. When a patient finally exhibits an acceptable antihypertensive response at a given dose level, no further dosage changes are made. The virtue of this approach is its theoretical similarity to clinical practice, and it allows an accurate overall estimate of the percentage of patients who can ultimately respond to a particular drug. It may also provide the most accurate within-patients dose-response curves (7).

The most obvious criticism of the titration design is that patients who reach the higher doses are, by definition, relative treatment failures. Not surprisingly, some studies using this type of design actually have reported greater efficacy at lower than at higher doses. This may be a common finding in hypertension where relatively high efficacy rates can occur at low doses. A potential solution to this problem is to undertake a "forced" titration in which patients continue to receive escalating doses even when lower doses are found to be efficacious. Although some critics might be concerned about the administration of potentially excessive doses, the risk to patients should be no greater than that which occurs in parallel group studies where patients can be directly randomized to treatment with the highest possible doses.

A further problem in studies employing multiple doses within each patient is the possibility of a time effect: when blood pressure is finally controlled by stepping up to a higher dose, it could be argued that the same desirable result could have been accomplished had the patient simply been allowed to remain at the previous dose level throughout the entire period. This type of error might explain why some of the older antihypertensive agents originally studied by titration methods, including such drugs as methyldopa, clonidine and hydrochlorothiazide, were recommended in doses far higher than are now considered necessary. A solution to this design problem would be to add a dose de-escalation phase to antihypertensive studies: it would be helpful to confirm the appropriateness of a particular dose by demonstrating that antihypertensive efficacy is lost when the dose is reduced.

DOSING INTERVALS

Much interest has focused on the question of dose intervals, for physicians and drug manufacturers have desired antihypertensive agents that are effective when administered just once or twice daily. Current FDA guidelines make two stipulations about documentation of a drug's duration of action. The first is that the drug produce a significantly greater decrement in blood pressure at the end of its dosing interval than placebo (administered in a parallel group of patients). Moreover, the FDA have suggested that the net drug effect (subtraction of placebo effect from total drug effect) should be "clinically meaningful". Recent experience suggests that this net effect should range between 3-6 mmHg.

The second FDA guideline is based on the relationship between peak and trough antihypertensive effects. By definition, the peak effect is the greatest decrement in blood pressure occurring during the dosing interval; this need not coincide with the pharmacokinetic peak. The trough, by definition, is the blood pressure effect measured at the end of the interdosing interval (regardless of whether or not the minimum clinical effect really occurs at that time). The crux of the FDA's recommendation is that the ratio of trough to peak (following subtraction of any placebo effect) should be between one-half to two-thirds.

This guideline has been motivated by concern that the duration of drug action may be extended inappropriately by the use of excessive dosage. Thus, a drug can be made to provide efficacy throughout the dosing interval at the price of a potentially dangerous early peak effect. Figure 1 shows the example of a study in which a drug was given in progressively increasing doses in order to accomplish significant effects at the end of its 24-hour dosing interval; it is evident that the maximum blood pressure effects a few hours after taking the drug are large, and that the trough-to-peak ratio correspondingly is small. Of course, ratios between effects do not readily represent clinical or even pharmacological events. Thus, the FDA have not required that these suggested ratios be achieved for approval of antihypertensive agents. Instead, it seems more rational to observe the criteria for peak and trough effects that are shown in Tables 1 and 2.

Table 1. Maximum Antihypertensive Response (Peak Effect)

1.	Does blood pressure rapidly fall to an excessively low level (below systolic of 90 mm Hg or diastolic of 50 mm Hg) in a meaningful number of patients?
2.	Are there any related adverse effects? --hypotension-dependent symptoms --evidence for myocardial ischemia (such as ECG changes)
3.	Are adverse events dose-related?

Table 2. Minimum Antihypertensive Response (Trough Effect)

1.	When compared with placebo treatment, is there a significant decrease in blood pressure?
2.	Is the overall response clinically meaningful?
3.	How does it compare with the efficacy of other antihypertensive agents?
4.	What percentage of patients exhibit strong responses such as a decrease of 10 mmHg in supine diastolic blood pressure?
5.	What percentage of patients have intermediate responses such as a decrease of 7 mm Hg or 4 mm Hg in supine diastolic blood pressure?

The Peak Effect

As shown in Table 1, the principal concern with peak effects is the possibility of adverse clinical reactions. As a practical issue, we suggest that reports of symptomatic side effects during clinical trials should state precisely the time of day at which they occurred, thereby making it possible to determine whether they reflect peak drug effects. This would appear to be a more precise method for establishing the clinical relevance of peak effects than depending, as is presently the case, on the relationship between the frequency of side effects and the size of the drug dose. It may be of value to search actively for evidence of clinical ill effects of excessive peak blood pressure decrements. It seems reasonable to ask: should such procedures as electrocardiograms or tests for orthostasis be performed in selected patients at the time of peak drug effects?

Trough Effects.

Is it relevant to consider trough effects in those patients who have failed to show any meaningful response to a drug? Should estimates of trough and peak, and the ratio between them, be carried out only in those patients who can be classified as responders? Because most clinicians usually check blood pressure effects at times close to the peak action of drugs, should we base measurements of trough and of trough:peak ratios only on those patients who exhibit clear peak effects?

Long-Term Studies.

Earlier we discussed the possibility that blood pressure effects of treatment may persist for weeks or months after discontinuation of previous drugs owing to the slow restoration of the underlying regulatory or structural mechanisms responsible for sustaining the clinical hypertension. As a converse of this argument, it could be suggested that optimum blood pressure effects might take several weeks or months to be established following the start of drug therapy. Moreover, once a drug has produced its effects on central mechanisms or perhaps on peripheral vascular tissues, smooth whole-day control of blood pressure might be maintained even if the drug does not act continuously throughout the 24-hour period. Thus, we should carry out peak and trough measurements not only after the customary 4-8 week period of study, but additionally after months of chronic treatment.

The Circadian Blood Pressure Pattern.

Blood pressure forms a clear pattern when measured throughout the day. Blood pressures at night are clearly lower than during the day, but rise sharply during the early to mid morning hours (9). This phenomenon is probably mediated through a sympathetically regulated arousal process, for plasma concentrations of norepinephrine and epinephrine appear to closely parallel the changes in blood pressure (10). The morning hours have attracted considerable attention, for a disproportionate frequency of such events as strokes and coronary episodes occurs at this time of day (11, 12). There is evidence that certain classes of antihypertensive agents, despite their excellent overall efficacy, may not adequately modify this potentially dangerous early morning blood pressure surge (13). Clearly, information concerning drug performance at different times of day (rather than just in relation to dosage time) would be of importance in characterizing antihypertensive agents. Vitally, with drugs that are administered once-daily, it may be just as important to measure their efficacy and duration of action when they are given as a nighttime dose as when they are given as the more traditional morning administration.

STUDIES OF DRUG COMBINATIONS

Fixed drug combinations have proved to be relatively unpopular with practicing clinicians, although manufacturers still continue to produce them. There appear to be two goals for fixed combinations of antihypertensive agents. The first is the traditional approach of adding a second drug to a patient whose blood pressure has failed to respond fully to an initial drug. The second, and newer goal, is to develop low dose fixed combinations that could be considered for initial therapy. A large proportion of patients ultimately require treatment with more than one drug, and it is a weakness of most drug development programs that inadequate data are obtained concerning the efficacy of the primary drug when given with other types of agents with which it is likely to be used in combination.

Low Dose Combinations.

Effective data require evaluation of efficacy of differing doses of each of the two drugs individually as well as their various combinations. The most powerful method for accomplishing this goal is to use a randomized parallel groups design comprising a matrix of cells representing each of the possible individual and combination treatments. Low dose combinations that potentially could be recommended for initial therapy of hypertension are only meaningful if the doses are at minimal levels (probably lower than the minimum effective doses for the drugs when given individually). It would also be helpful, although not essential, to show some type of synergy between the drugs; that is, to demonstrate that a low dose of one of the drugs can significantly shift to the left the dose response curve of the other.

Addition Studies.

Most studies of drug combinations have been carried out in circumstances where an initial drug has been unsuccessful in decreasing blood pressure adequately. The second drug is then added and titrated to its most effective dose. However, it is never certain that the combination is truly necessary in such patients, for the efficacy accomplished by the combination may be due entirely to the action of the second drug alone. Thus, in best characterizing two drugs it would seem desirable to test each agent individually as well as in combination. This is the basis for crossover studies that recently have been recommended as providing more statistical power, with a need for fewer patients, than traditional combination studies (14).

Such studies need not be carried out only in patients found to have resistance to treatment (which can be a rather expensive and tedious process), but can be planned from the beginning as a randomized sequence crossover design that will examine each drug individually, as well as the combination, in every patient. To add validity to this approach, there should be a placebo washout period between each of the treatment periods. This type of research should not be used solely for the development of fixed combinations, but should be used to more broadly characterize interactions between the primary drug and other antihypertensive agents with which it is likely to be used in combination.

Duration Studies.

Interactions between drugs can not only enhance the amplitudes of the blood pressure effects, but may also prolong them. It is possible that drugs might alter each other's pharmacokinetic properties. A recent study, for example, has shown that a low dose of diuretic can substantially prolong the duration of action of an ACE inhibitor (15). It may also be important to check peak and trough measurements when drugs are given in combination, for there can be a danger of excessive peak blood pressure reductions.

REFERENCES

1. Report by the Management Committee. Lancet. 1:1261-1267, 1988.
2. Drayer, J.I.M., Weber M.A. Hypertension. 5:180-113, 1983.
3. Pickering, T.G., James, G.D., Bodie, C., Harshfield, G.A., Black, S., Laragh, J.H. JAMA. 259:225-228, 1988.
4. Weber, M.A., Cheung, D.G., Graettinger, W.F., Lipson, J.L. JAMA. 259:3281-5, 1988.
5. Sammelsson, O., Wilmhelmsen, L., Anderson, O.K., Pennert, K., Berglund, G. JAMA. 285:1768-1776, 1987.
6. Graettinger, W.F., Lipson, J.L., Klein, R.C., Cheung, D.G., Weber, M.A. Chest. 96:74-79, 1989.
7. Sheiner, L.B., Beal, S.L., Sambol, N.C. Clin. Pharmacol. Ther. 46:63-77, 1989.
8. Guyatt, G., Sackett, D., Adachi, J., Roberts, R., Chong, J., Rosenbloom, D., Keller, D. Can. Med. Assoc. J. 139:497-503, 1988.
9. Weber, M.A., Drayer, J.I.M., Nakamura, D.K., Wyle, F.A. Am. J. Cardiol. 54:115-119, 1984.
10. Linsell, C.R., Lightman, S.L., Mullen, P.E., Brown, M.J., Causon, R.C. J. Clin. Endocrinol. Metab. 60:1210-5, 1985.
11. Agnoli, A., Manfredi, M., Mossuto, L., Piccinelli, A. Rev. Neurol. 131:597-606, 1975.
12. Myers, A., Dewar, H.A. Br. Heart. J. 37:1133-43, 1975.
13. Raftery, E.B., Carrageta, M.O. Int. J. Cardiol. 7:337-346, 1985.
14. Menard, J., Serrurier, D., Bautier P., Plovin P.F., Corvol, P. Hypertension. 11:153-9, 1988.
15. Cheung, D.G., Gasster, J.L., Weber, M.A. Arch. Intern. Med. 149:2021-2025, 1989.

6

HOW DOES ONE DEFINE DOSE-DURATION OF AN ANTIHYPERTENSIVE DRUG? WHAT IS THE ROLE OF NON-MEM AND THE PEAK/THROUGH MEASUREMENT?

Raymond J. Lipicky, M.D.

Director, Division of Cardio-renal Drug Products
FOOD AND DRUG ADMINISTRATION
Rockville, MD 20857

For a new drug to gain approval for the therapy of hypertension it is necessary but perhaps not sufficient that there be two or more adequately controlled trials that demonstrate an antihypertensive effect in a general population of patients with essential hypertension, and that the dosing interval for the antihypertensive effect be clear. The antihypertensive effect is taken simply as a reflection of a change in blood pressure in comparison to placebo. One could do a positive controlled trial which would be harder to do as a study because you have to be sure of the correct dose. Alternate possibilities to consider are baseline control with reversal or randomized withdrawal with placebo.

The general population criterion implies a few things. The first thing that people emphasize is that hypertension is multifactorial and thus a reasonably large sample is required. It isn't too hard to tell that an agent is an antihypertensive agent in a sample of two people, but that clearly will be inadequate to demonstrate that it could be useful in a general population. Most physicians choose to treat individuals for hypertension based on cuff blood pressure measured in the office. The development of an antihypertensive drug assumes that the blood pressure is predictive of future events, so blood pressure measured by cuff is often considered the prime endpoint. That doesn't mean one can't measure other things to derive insights into the pathophysiology of hypertension. But, cuff blood pressure measurements need to be a part of the criteria for selecting patients and, in fact, one would want to have blood pressure measured in more than one position.

Effects on blood pressure need to be demonstrated at the interdosing intervals, primarily based on the idea that since blood pressure is being accepted as a surrogate for clinical endpoints related to the natural history of hypertension that have been shown using drugs that have long-duration reactions, there ought to be some antihypertensive effect for the entire dosing interval.

The second reason for knowing about the interdosing interval is to evaluate the trade-off between side effects and the dosing interval. The probabilities of being able to demonstrate a drug effect as it is related to dose is highest if one looks at the peak effect, and least if one looks at the trough effect. If one did a trial and looked at the relationship between the dose and effect by measuring blood pressure only at trough, there may be practically no dose related effect measurable even though at peak there is a prominent dose related effect. That may also in fact be true for side effects, although in general side effects are not collected from the vantage point of being able to draw those kinds of differentiations.

In terms of design issues, if one uses a conventional placebo versus drug design where the drug is titrated, it is now clear that one derives no information with respect to dose-related effects when traditional methods are used for data analysis. Crossover designs could lead to useful information, but basically one would have to treat for long periods of time in each leg and that becomes impractical. The parallel fixed dose design has a major defect in that it does not tell one how to change doses in any individual patient, so each of these traditional designs can be useful for some things and fail with respect to other considerations.

A newer design is the factorial design where not only can one get information related to dose response for individual drugs, but also for drug combinations. Another is to use the forced titration placebo controlled trial, but analyse the data not according to conventional means, but according to techniques that have been discussed by Dr. Scheiner and Beil using mixed-effects-modeling and a particular computer program called Non-Mem which can extract useful dose response information that is pertinent to individuals from group data. The factorial design and Non-Mem analysis involve the use of model dependent analyses. Statisticians and biologists, generally, shy away from model dependant analysis with respect to hypothesis testing. So, newer approaches also have some advantages and disadvantages.

If one is willing to accept the fact that for almost any drug there is some kind of dose-effect relationship, and recognize that over the course of a 24-hour day that untreated blood pressure has systematic variability and that superimposed on that variability is a drug effect, and if what one wants to do is to insure that the duration of drug effect is clear, then one has to be able to pull out of the data the drug effect so that the shape of the curve can be appreciated not only in an individual, but in a population. A tall order, but clearly, one needs to measure blood pressure more than once a day.

If one measures the blood pressure so that one can estimate the peak, and through effects, our attitude is that generally speaking (if side effects appear to be related to dose) that if more than 50% of the blood pressure effect is lost in the dosing interval, that dosing interval is a nonviable. However, if the drug beats placebo at the dosing interval and if side effects are not dose related, then it may be acceptable to have lost more than 50% of the effect. These kinds of comparisons are pretty arbitrary.

It would be nicer if one were able to characterize the shape of the blood pressure curve in some mathematical way and make blood pressure a function of time, and be able to find a function that fits the data and be able to express the findings in terms of probabilities that the blood pressure diurnal shape has been altered significantly by drug. Obviously such methodology has not been well developed, and there are a variety of people that are currently studying such methods and exploring their applicability.

Within the context of this meeting, current antihypertensive guidelines accept blood pressure as the measure of clinical efficacy and emphasize description of the effects of an antihypertensive in terms of dose and dose-interval. Although a relatively easy to measure variable is of primary interest, significant methodological problems make description of effects challenging and force a number of choices that produce answers to different questions but no single approach answers all relevant questions.

PANEL ON HYPERTENSION METHODOLOGY

Dr. Morganroth: Dr. Lipicky states that he still considers the measurement from the cuff as the critical endpoint measurement that has been correlated best with benefit, but we also heard from both Drs. White and Weber that the ambulatory blood pressure monitor data correlated better with vascular endpoints. In fact, many apparent hypertensives in the office are not really hypertensive by 24-hour monitoring when one looks at the cuff blood pressure, in fact, that group tends not to be responsive to antihypertensive drugs perhaps because they are really not hypertensive and if one has a problem with variability of data perhaps the 24-hour data is better.

Dr. Lipicky: I need to clarify my comment. I don't know that blood pressure measured by the cuff is important or valid or a predictor or tells anybody anything. I think what I was saying was that in the process of drug development the data that is collected should have predictive value, and that predictive value is with respect to how it would be used in practice. In practice people measure the blood pressure with a cuff and make decisions with respect to whether or not to treat by that method. Thefore, a development program should contain that informtion because that is what is trying to be predicted. Now clearly from the advantage point of science and research it ought to contain other measurements, but if it contains all the other measurements and did not contain cuff blood pressure measurements it wouldn't be fullfilling predicted roles as I see it.

Dr. Alexander: In follow-up to Dr. Lipicky's comments, that would seem to be true for all the other things we are now doing in terms of peak-trough and dosing interval. A lot of those things are not really validated in the sense that the initial trials were showing mortality improvements. They did not worry about the blood pressure at the trough level. They did not look at the 24-hour blood pressure curve. So, I agree with you in terms of the blood pressure cuff, but a lot of the other issues addressed in those studies didn't conform to the current standards either.

<u>Dr. Lipicky:</u> Again, just to clarify my comments. My comments are not related to that, that is the idea of looking at peak and trough as a means of getting at dose response information and dose interval information. This is something that is necessary to adequately describe the pharmacodynamic action of the drug, and intelligently decide whether the dose and dose interval that are being recommended are, in fact, reasonable. Those decisions have nothing to do with whether or not the cuff blood pressure has predictive value with respect to morbitity or mortality. The idea of being satisfied with measuring blood pressure or some parameter associated with blood pressure has to do with the idea of morbitity or mortality in accepting that it will change the blood pressure, and accepts that as a surrogate. That, in fact, is the equivalent having described the benefit. So the two ideas are totally unrelated.

<u>Dr. Pickering:</u> I would like to seriously suggest that we dispense with the cuff measurement as a requirement. I think what some of us are saying is that it's necessary but not sufficient. However, whether we should look at people who had consistently elevated clinic pressures, and perhaps some of the other measurements as well and I would certainly like to see studies in which the entry criteria included not only an elevated clinic pressure, but either an elevated ambulatory pressure in addition or in some cases left ventricular hypertrophy depending on the purpose of the study.

<u>Dr. Temple:</u> The point of most trials is to see where the blood pressure falls. It really doesn't matter whether it's the relevant blood pressure on the whole or whether you can get a more refined measure and exclude variability. But the question is whether changes in cuff blood pressure in a placebo controlled trial demonstrate that a drug can lower the blood pressure, and of course they can. The question was what is the most relevant blood pressure cuff to survival. In a different form there is no reason to think that any one of those measurements doesn't tell you whether the drug is active.

The idea that you should have 24-hour controlled blood pressure comes from the observation that the earliest trials that did show improved survival were drugs that had very little duration and action. In the original trials, I read that placebo three times a day was probably not necessary. But in any event, the drugs that were given surely achieved 24-hours of control, which means they were still there and active after 24-hours, and that is the major theoretical reason that we insist that any regimen proposed control blood pressure in 24-hours. We don't know that this is necessary, but we know that the trials have been done.

Dr. Weber raised a point that we perhaps assume that the drug is still active at 24-hours and it is morning before the next dose, then it was probably active right up to that point. I suppose that it is possible that a beta-blocker in the middle of the night does not really do much, maybe that is something that needs to be thought about. That's why we have trough data that were taken as evidence of round the clock therapy. Of course, we did not have 24-hour values when that was devised.

<u>Dr. White:</u> I've made an observation that the timing of the trough measurement is relatively crucial. If somebody is going to decide to see the patient before they go to work for a trough measurement at 7 A.M., you may see very little effect versus 3 or 4 hours later when their sympathetic nervous system was going. You might see a greater differential just as it was pointed out on that 48-hour study, so perhaps we could have been making a mistake for a couple years by saying all these peak trough studies should be designed so that when the patients come in between 8 and 10 A.M. or between 7 and 9 A.M. they should be dose. Why not dose them at noon, 24-hours later when the drug probably is going to have activity because of the resistance.

<u>Dr. Temple:</u> Let's say that the drug pharmacokinetically is a 24-hour drug. That is you can show that 24-hours after that it is still there and still has its effect, but suppose it turns out that the previous 4-hours it does not do alot. What do we do?

<u>Dr. White</u> I think that is a very important issue, because if you look at the hours between 2 A.M. and 6 A.M. in which the patient is sleeping and the blood pressure is at the slowest point of the day and in mild hypertension sometimes there are varied levels, 110/60. I don't think that there is any good evidence at this point in time that it is worth

lowering that blood pressure any further. Lowering blood pressure too low could have a damaging effect on the heart. There have been enough cross sectional studies now that do suggest that that lowering of elevated blood pressure at night could potentially be harmful. Not showing an effect between 2 a.m. and 6 a.m. does not bother me in the least.

Dr. Weber: I'd like to get back to the point that the aim of trials so far has showed that drugs can lower blood pressure. Trials have shown that at least we can prevent strokes, and this can be done regardless of what treatment we use or whether it is shorter acting or how it is administered. One of the thinks we have to confront is the fact that we have not done a tremendously good job in treating hypertension in regards to preventing coronary events. I think a good amount of research is now ongoing away from the therapeutic area. Lowering blood pressure seems to help in severe hypertensives who are prone to strokes or prone to heart failure or renal insufficiency, but most of our patients are going to get coronary events and die from the complications of those and we have not done a great job in this area.

Dr. Cohn: There is no question that the lowering of blood pressure in a subset of 60 million people in this country that have hypertension has a long-term impact on morbitity and mortality. I think we would all agree that all 60 million people with high blood pressure are not at risk for premature morbitity or mortality because of their blood pressure elevation. So their blood pressure is useful in a population way and certainly useful at certain high levels in an individual way of predicting morbitity and mortality but it is clearly not a specific marker for the patient who has a high risk of morbitity or mortality. It is also true that in terms of lowering blood pressure the conventional wisdom is appropriate and that is that a drug which will lower blood pressure effectively throughout the 24-hours with minimal side effects is the ideal agent to utilize and it would be nice to demonstrate that the drug you are using if it's aim is to lower blood pressure is producing its desired effect throughout the course of the day, but that is a totally different agenda than the issue about what the relationship is between blood pressure's morbid events and how to select the appropriate patient to treat. It is also true that there are a large number of people who are so called normal hypertensives who are not being exposed to antihypertensive drugs who are at very high risk of premature morbitity and mortality and they are not now being treated because we are not identifying them because we are basing our screening and our management entirely on the measurement of systolic and diastolic pressures which vary throughout the day and it is different when asleep and awake, etc.

It seems to me that the other agenda is to clearly address the issue as to what should be an appropriate surrogate for vascular abnormality that leads to hypertension, which in itself may accelarate the vascular abnormality but is not necessarily a marker for the presence of the vascular abnormality, and I don't know what that marker is yet, I suggest that they are many others that we're going to be addressing over the years to come. But, until we identify that, I think we are sort of playing games with a number that isn't itself a very specific or sensitive marker for the presence of vascular abnormality. That's not quite the same for drug development. I have a feeling that in 20 years down the road that we will not be looking at drugs for their effect on blood pressure alone but will be administering drugs in an effort to prevent progression of vascular abnormalities that lead to premature morbitity and mortality in our society.

Dr. Morganroth: It appears that most of the members of this panel feels that the cuff blood pressure is becoming archaic because of its insensitivity. In drug development in addition to having some studies identifying patients with cuff measurements to copy current clinical practice, there needs to be some other measurement beyond the casual cuff data such as 24-hour blood pressure monitoring data. We need to look at pressure for a 24-hour duration, actual individual responsiveness, dose relationship in individual patients, etc.

Dr. Temple: It really all depends on what you want to do with it. You can learn whether a drug lowers blood pressure by cuff measurement; you can do the cuff measurements at more than one time. That way you can learn what the hour by hour characteristics of the drug are. I think it is pretty clear that people are interested in that. You really do want to know if the drug is producing a 30mm trough at some point of the day and a 5mm trough at the end. That may be evidence that you are using the wrong dose interval. It may mean that you want to tell people that that's going on.

A single blood pressure taken casually at some time in the day has not been okay for a long time. For a while it was at the end of the 24-hour value. Then we figured out that peak effect was worth something, so now it's at least a rough peak value and a trough value, and it's probably moving to the point where at least some of the data on 24-hour effects are now appearing all the time.

The other questions that were raised are what is meaningful, what corresponds to morbitity or mortality and there we are in the dark. What you want to do is identify the differences between drugs and the way they effect some measures, but we are some distance from that. You could compare outcomes in drugs that have one effect or another if you are prepared to give drugs to 10,000 patients.

Dr. Pickering: I really don't think we should give the impression that cuff pressure is archaic and should be thrown out. If we through it out we are then lost, because while these new measurements may be more sensitive we really don't have the data relating to either ambulatory pressure or left ventricular mass or any other measure in terms of prognosis and treatment effects. It's more a question of supplementing the cuff presures, and I think the emphasis is going to be on stratifying patients with elevated cuff pressures to try and pick out who among that large population is at low risk or high risk and I think this is where these new meausures are going to be helpful.

Dr. Lipicky: I think that if you look at the current draft of the hypertensive guidelines the difference that exists in those compared with what exists in the past was to be able to get a better description of drug effect. Indeed, get a better description of drug effect so one can acquire different kinds of measurements and, in fact, figure out how to handle those things in some reasonable way and what means of handling those measurements is predictive and is useful, and all of this is unknown. At least from the advantage point of guidelines the demand is being made.

Dr. Morganroth: Another question is how much data are necessary? Can one obtain data from a 12-patient study and to blood pressure is well characterized blood pressure, but have 98% of the efficacy data based on casual blood pressure without having it in a large
population? How much dose duration data do we need?

Dr. Lipicky: By casual do you mean being sometimes standard cuff blood pressure?

Dr. Morganroth: Yes.

Dr. Lipicky: The data have to be at the interdosing interval. In fact; if at the interdosing interval one does not have a antihypertensive effect then the discussion sort of stops. If that is there, then the discussion begins. The degree to which all of these other kinds of things are addressed remains a poorly definied entity. How well one defines that the side effects are dose related is clearly important because if you have all the peak effect

data you want but you don't know how side effects are related to dose and you have a difficult time discussing this data. So I don't think there is a single answer to the question you asked.

Dr. Cody: I just want to add to some information that has been said. Those people who have blood pressure either at one time frame of the day or for 24-hours day, does not eliminate the possibility that there is a vascular abnormality present in all of us or some fraction of all of us. I think those are two different issues and I think it would be quite an action trying to look at not only drug responses for FDA related issues, but physiological issues.

Dr. Cohn: Let me propose to Dr. Lipicky a hypothetical situation. Suppose a drug, which was a specific inhibitor of vascular growth, was developed and administered to a group of mild to moderate hypertensives in a long-term trial and there was absolutely no effect on blood pressure but there was a striking reduction in morbitity and mortality from vascular disease. How would you deal with that drug?

You are not trying to lower the blood pressure, that is not the treatment for hypertension, you are trying to prevent vascular morbid events. I do believe that vascular growth is important to the progression of these processes, and if you can inhibit it without lowering the blood pressure you might have a happier patient with fewer events. How will that require a reassessment of our goal to lower blood pressure as a major therapeutic goal?

Dr. Lipicky: At the moment those things are handled separately as to save lives in patients with congestive heart failure. The data as you described it would be to save lives of people with hypertension not a therapy of hypetension per se.

Dr. Cohn: If a drug company came to you before the end of phase two and said look this drug doesn't lower blood pressure but we want to test it in hypertensives, you might try to discourage them.

Dr. Temple: Maybe not. Do you mean on ethical grounds because it's not safe to leave hypertensives untreated?

Dr. Cohn: Well no just based on what Ray said a moment ago that if the blood pressure isn't lowered you would discourage the dosing regimen from being employed.

Dr. Lipicky: I don't know about that, that's different. I suppose any trial has to have some reasonable scientific basis or otherwise you get into the problems of ethics. There has to be some rationale to serve as the basis for the hypothesis that is tested by the trial, otherwise you get into the ethical portion. That does come-up in discussion once in a while. If there was some reason to believe that mortality would be effected without effecting blood pressure.

Dr. Temple: It seems to me that things like that have happened. Everybody knows the main problem with heart failure was that the heart was not beating strong enough until some people came up with some other explanations of what was going on. The most totally irrational way of speeding heart failure was by lowering resistence.

Dr. Kaplan: If I were a drug company trying to offer a hypertensive drug today, the first that I would require was that they get rid all of the office hypertensives from their studies. It is clear that that's going to diminished the apparent effectiveness of the given drug. If the drug companies are willing to do that, and all of the patients who have had ambulatory blood pressure monitoring as their entry into this trial to exclude those who are out of the office hypertensive, will you except their NDA because clearly they are going to exclude a lot of patients who today will be treated for hypertension?

Dr. Temple: They would just eliminate the people who don't have the disease. Actually, there have been various attempts to do that. If you have office hypertension, how come it goes away the first time you're in the randomized part of the trial? The very first measurement in a randomized trial is always 5 or 6 mm lower. But people have often had prolonged periods of single blind placebo to try to eliminate these things and look for stability during that period and if you do it right, sometimes you don't see much of a change on a placebo.

Dr. White: I think that an opposite situation could occur as well. Sometimes when you do 24-hour blood pressure studies on these patients who have apparently high-normal blood pressures in the clinic setting and you have elevated blood pressures out of the office. This would be classified as a sustained hypertensive, and if you did not do this study you would miss them and you would end up putting them on therapy unappropriately. So it could go either way as the only unbiased methodology that can be used in defining the hypertension patient in one of these studies.

Dr. Alexander: We've had a lot of experience trying to use ambulatory blood pressure in multicenter clinical trials, and that was not a happy episode.

Dr. Pickering: I would like to make a comment about this repeated clinic measurement for improving the selection of patients. It is certainly true with repeated clinic measurements you will tend to get lower readings. There was one study that showed you needed 6 visits before the pressure plateaus, but even then there are still patients who will have persistently elevated clinic pressures but normal pressures outside the clinic. There was an interesting study, which I think hasn't been published yet which was done in Norway. They screened young men and they picked out the ones who had the highest pressures on screening and then they divided them into two groups and they sent them different letters. One of them was told that your pressure is high and you need to come back and have it rechecked and another was just told we want to remeasure your pressure. Although the two groups had identical pressures on the first screening, however, when they rechecked them there was a 15mm of mercury difference between the two which persisted throughout the testing procedure which lasted 45 minutes. So I think one can get into major problems with this type of procedure. And this is where the ambulatory readings are helpful.

Dr. Morganroth: I assume the one with the 15mm increase was the group that was suppose to have high blood pressure?

Dr. Pickering: Yes, that is right.

Dr. Weber: It is becoming apparent that hypertension is a kind of a syndrome which does include having a high blood pressure, but also has some other specific abnormalities that are not just their by chance. It seems to be inherented along with the propensity behind blood pressure and the growing studies have shown that lipid abnormalities or LDL binding characteristics are the difference in hypertensive patients in what vascular abnormalities occur. In children we can find early evidence for diastolic dysfunction of the left ventricle well before these kids become hypertensive. Before we can release a drug or describe it adequately, do we really need to know its effect on cholesterol, insulin, glucose, or vascular changes?

Dr. Temple: You do have to characterize the effects that a drug has on other relative systems so that you will at least need a measure of lipids for most of these drugs. It isn't even that we demand them it's that there are potential claims or borderline claims that are there. Certainly an interesting question could be increasing the effect on LV dysfunction and on hypertrophy. I think you will see more characterization of those effects in time. The nervousness I have is that it is easy to focus on the latest fad and forget some of the things that went before. If you watch the current advertising, the calcium channel blockers you can already see this. There is a lot of focus on what they don't do and it would be easy to forget that they have never been shown to lower rate of strokes or improve survival in any situation known to man in contrast to beta-blockers which have some effects that are perceived as adverse and yet in the post-infarction setting are clearly more successful than calcium channel blockers. How much long-term safety data in general are required for these kinds of drugs? In the past is has been essentially short-term data. Have you given any thought to how much long-term safety data is necessary?

Dr. Lipicky: Yes. We have a guideline, but I guess it is fair to say the answer to Dr. Morganroth's question is no.

Dr. Temple: To learn what the adverse consequence of 5% increase in cholesterol is the test for several NIHs since it is going to require thousands of patients. Those things are not easily accessable. You can make a guess which is probably not good. You have to look at the effects of all of these agents and in the end large-scale trials are the only answer.

Dr. Morganroth: Are they required preapproval?

Dr. Temple: The trials I have in mind strike me as beyond a resonable capacity of any individual drug company. Whether they are in the capacity of the country is another issue.

Dr. Morganroth: Why is a year's worth of long-term data not sufficient for approvability for a good base for a program?

Dr. Temple: That is about what it is. It might be up to 500. You are talking about the attempts to try and find organ toxicity. I think we don't have any illusion that you are going to find that kind of effect. It certainly seems like something to discuss and we would be happy to take suggestions, but it does not seem accessible to the kinds of trials that can be done.

Dr. Cohn: In reference to the issue of LVH, suppose a drug company has a new compound that seems to be a good antihypertensive and as part of their studies they compare it with an ACE inhibitor over a 6 month period of time, and at the end of the trial the two drugs are equally effective in lowering blood pressure but the ACE inhibitors has reversed LVH and this new drug has not. Would that be a safety concern, would it be approvable but with a warning in the labeling or would it be disregarding completely in the labeling?

Dr. Temple: It could go in the clinical pharmacology section.

Dr. Lipicky: I think not.

Dr. Temple: That is something we would like to take advice on, but probably beta-blockers are not as good at producing LVH as some other drugs. What does that tell you? They are good for post-infarction use; they help in some people with coronary artery disease.

Dr. Kaplan: There has been certainly a lot of data presented this morning that suggested that LVH is bad for you. At least there is a relationship between the presence of LVH and morbidity and mortality. However, we have not proved that controlling LVH is good for you and I guess that is the issue. Until you can demonstrate that then you can't really include that in your approval.

Dr. Lipicky: It raises a bunch of interesting issues in terms of labeling. On the one hand I think I would like to argue the point that any information that can easily be described about the drug belongs on the label. The problem is that when one does that it begins to be used in promotion and not reasonably. Consequently my biases are that if you really don't know what that thing means, it doesn't belong in the labeling.

Dr. Temple: However, we are not perfectly consistent in that. Inderal, I know says that resting cardiac output is not impaired compared to other drugs. That's true. It's not known to be of great importance but since it was true it is in their label. There are some true not clearly relevant things that do appear in labeling.

Dr. Lipicky: They are very difficult decisions to make because they are not based on whether or not the data is good or bad. They are not based on whether or not one thinks that the labeling information will be misused from the advantage point of representing the drug in promotion.

Dr. Temple: Sometimes what you try to do does not really work.

Dr. Kaplan: The fact that people who make Pindolol have been bragging about the fact that it does not reduce cardiac output, I don't consider that a problem but they have done a poor job of selling the drug. The fact is that there has not been that effect compared to other beta-blockers. It seems to me that they would have to talk about that, and the fact that it is in the product labeling and you're saying that that is giving them an edge in someway I don't look upon it that way at all. I think that's the sort of information that the world should know about. The fact that it hasn't been a selling point for that drug maybe doctors realize that doesn't matter whether it effects cardiac output at all in the long run.

Dr. Temple: Obviously we thought that it was true and it ought to be in there too which is why we allowed it. However, when you learn about it from advertising you don't learn that most of the problems with cardiac output is probably in an exercise situation where just like everyother drug you probably don't worry about this hasn't been correlated with fatigue, depression or anything known to be of importance. If one were sure that the whole thing were balanced one would be more comfortable about dropping these things in labeling. But, of course, it is hard to ask that of someone who's advertising.

Dr. Pickering: I want to make a comment about blood pressure variability. In fact, most estimates suggest that mearly because you have more readings in a ambulatory recording you can actually reduce the variability of measures on repeated occassions as compared with the clinic measurements. Jim Conway, in Oxford, has shown when you are doing a calculation for the number of subjects you need in a clinical trial to show a treatment effect of a drug because of the improved reproducability of ambulatory measures you usually need a smaller sample providing it is done right.

Dr. Weber: I would like to make a technical point in response to that. Since his original study was done with over 400 patients I think the manufacturers of the automated monitoring equipment have gone through at least three new generations of devices and more recently I think even inexperienced investigators are getting very reliable data.

Dr. White: Furthermore, to add to that there is a variety of helpers in the field these days to help the pharmaceutical industry. You can't really expect an inexperienced investigator to perform these studies adequately without some formal training session.

Dr. Morganroth: If you were going to define the two well controlled trials you need to establish approvability with a new antihypertensive drug what would be the basic design of those two trials?

Dr. Lipicky: That's a very difficult question to answer because it is necessitates laying out a whole program. If one wanted to provide the absolute barest minimum of controlled trial information that said that interdosing interval drug be placebo, it would be placebo versus titration. Now whether that would be an economical thing to do considering all of the other information that is necessary to obtain is unclear. I could think of better ways of spending money to get more information. If the question is what is the minimum amount of information that would be required to make it possible would be a placebo controlled drug.

Dr. Frishman: If you had data presented to you comparing two different antihypertensive agents, one showing greater blood pressure lowering efficacy than another, with the data that is now available about lowering blood pressure too much may be dangerous. Would you say that the more effective antihypertensive drug was a better drug? Was the question in fact that there may be a potential danger of lowering the blood pressure too much? How will we look at this in the future?

Dr. Lipicky: For me to answer that question you will have to provide a little more information. Appropriate doses of each drug were used and it wasn't because of some known demographic issue. By all available information you could really say one lowered blood pressure more than the other.

Dr. Frishman: Then you could make the observation that one drug worked better at lowering the blood pressure.

Dr. Temple: Someone treating a hypertensive patient has on what ever basis some goal of blood pressure that he is trying to reach. Some people don't reach it with one drug, and it's probably better to have a drug that is more powerful than the other. That is one alternative to adding another drug that might be desirable.

Dr. Lipicky: We would need more information than you are providing. If the only thing that you know is that it is more effective than that's good for approval, and basically current labeling unless it is likely that the drug is less effective or has a very small effect doesn't really mention active effect because they are titrated.

Dr. Temple: You have that sort of thing all the time. Beta-blockers are better than diuretics and the reverse. If the question is what do you need to show that your drug is an active antihypertensive agent you could even set up the study by using two lower doses of the other drug. All of those things would be evidence that the drug is active. Now if differences were very small and there was no placebo it might be hard for us to say what kind of magnitude of effect you would have.

Dr. Morganroth: Mike Weber mentioned that combination data would be required to affiliate the drug. It that currently the policy?

Dr. Lipicky: It is usually required in some fashion or another that a new chemical entity is studied in combination with something. More or less it may be loosely constructed in that an individual has received two drugs at the same time and nothing bad happened. Generally speaking having found out whether in combination it requires different dose or whether in combination there are different kinds of side effects or that sort of business from the advantage point of a systematic study that's generally missing. I think it is an oversight at how people allocate resources in the development of an antihypertensive drug because it would be impossible to satisfy some of that more effectively and to get new drugs aporoved and some combination drugs approved to save money. It's not common and it really is a matter of how one wants to allocate resources.

Dr. Alexander: I think most companies look at the safety of the different combinations of therapies and the increase in side effects. The issue is what drugs do you want studied together?

Dr. Weber: I did not have any specific in mind except there are now 5 or 6 classes of antihypertensive agents and a lot of doctors are eventually going to try to mix and match all of them in an attempt to get efficacy. I am looking at it not just from a safety point of view but from a therapeutic opportunity point of view. I think while doing some of the work that we did looking at the ace inhibitor with the diurectic showed that not only did they work well together but there was a shift in the dose response in the presence of one drug dose response curve of the another drug also. Is some cases this was quite dramatic.

Dr. Temple: It is very common for the interactions with diuretics to be explored for non-diuretic antihypertensive agents, most of them come in with at least some study. Sometimes the major studies are carried out in the major dose response study. What other kinds of combinations would you look at, are some that we should add routinely. Should everything now be studied along with ACE inhibitors?

Dr. Weber: I think their ought to be some information. I think a lot of physicians have picked up on the fact that ACE inhibitors and calcium blockers are a very effective combination. I think this is a popular from of treatment especially for physicians who don't like to treat with diuretics. However, doctors who do start their patients on an ACE inhibitor might now add a calcium blocker as the second-line drug.

Dr. Temple: That probably would have not made since even a year ago when there was hardly any proof, now that it is growing in use it makes sense.

Dr. Lipicky: In general, there is information in respect to more than a new chemical entity. There is information, but is not necessarily systematic, and it is more oriented towards safety than it is along the lines of demonstrating that two in combination are more effective than either one alone or that one can give a smaller dose of one in the presence of another. To accomplish those ends the two are more effective together than either one alone or that you can change the dose of one. This really requires more than a small study because those are not easy end to accomplish generally, at least the ones that we have seen tried. So it comes down to whether what you are suggesting is that there be systematic study of more than one other agent or that the experiential data that currently is included is sufficient.

Dr. Temple: I don't think there is anything really convincing data that show the dose response is any different if you start at the same blood pressure.

Dr. Lipicky: They are occasional circumstances where patients responses are exagerated.

Dr. Temple: I am convinced that beta-blockers don't have as big of an effect as ACE inhibitors. In a parallel dose response curve it is usual to titrate the dose to the higher dose and not to put people on the full dose immediately, so that while you are doing parallel dose response study you also have the opportunity to do a dose titration, in a forced titration kind of study. Since you have a parallel placebo group that's a reasonable source of data in which you can look at individual response.

II. WHAT SHOULD BE REQUIRED FOR FDA APPROVABILITY OF A NEW ANTIHYPERTENSIVE DRUG?

7

What Have We Learned from Prior Clinical Trials of Antihypertensive Drug Therapy?

Aram V. Chobanian, M.D.

Clinical trials performed during the past three decades have provided valuable data regarding the effects of antihypertensive drug therapy on the development of cardiovascular complications. The data differ somewhat according to the degree of severity of hypertension, and the findings in patients with moderate and severe hypertension (diastolic blood pressures 105-114 mmHg and $\geq$ 115 mmHg, respectively) should best be considered separately from those in patients with mild hypertension (diastolic pressures 90-104 mmHg).

In patients with moderate and severe hypertension, impressive benefits from blood pressure lowering are well documented and include reductions in total mortality as well as in incidence of hemorrhagic and thrombotic strokes, congestive heart failure, renal failure, dissecting aneurysms, left ventricular hypertrophy, and progression in severity of hypertension. These complications of hypertension appear related directly to blood pressure elevation and would be expected to be affected favorably by blood pressure lowering. The benefits of treatment in moderate and severe hypertensives appear to be independent of gender, race, or age. It remains uncertain whether differences exist between antihypertensive drugs in their ability to prevent complications in patients with moderate or severe hypertension since the clinical trials to date have involved use of combined drug therapy with diuretic, sympatholytic and vasodilator drugs.

Clinical trials in patients with mild hypertension have demonstrated favorable effects of drug treatment on the development of stroke, left ventricular hypertrophy, and progression in severity of hypertension. However, the effects on total mortality and on myocardial infarction and other complications of coronary heart disease have been uncertain.

Failure to reduce complications related to atherosclerotic vascular disease in mild hypertensives remains a major problem. Several hypotheses have been forwarded to explain this failure. These have included the possibility that deleterious effects of treatment might offset any favorable influence of blood pressure lowering. The induction of serum lipid and glucose tolerance abnormalities by certain diuretics and beta blockers and of hypokalemia and cardiac arrhythmias by thiazide diuretics has been cause for concern. The frequent failure to control co-existing cardiovascular risk factors that affect the progression of atherosclerosis and its complications has also been considered by some to be a factor. In addition, there has been recent concern that excessive lowering of blood pressure (e.g. less than 85 mmHg diastolic) might be detrimental to myocardial perfusion in some patients with mild hypertension and might predispose to the development of myocardial infarction. However, although all of these hypotheses deserve further exploration, relatively little direct evidence exists as yet to indicate conclusively the involvement of any of these factors.

Several classes of effective antihypertensive drugs are currently available, but comparisons between them in long-term trials of mild hypertension have been limited. Most clinical trials utilized diuretic-based treatment initially, but recently, some of them involved beta blockers as well. In the Medical Research Council study, bendroflumethazide, propranolol, and placebo therapy were compared. Both drugs reduced the incidence of stroke significantly but neither significantly affected total mortality or the development of coronary heart disease. Little difference was also noted between diuretic and beta blocker-treated groups in the Heart Attack Primary Prevention in Hypertension study. In contrast, in the Metoprolol Atherosclerosis Prevention in Hypertensives trial, metoprolol therapy was associated with a much lower incidence of total mortality and both fatal and non-fatal myocardial infarction than diuretic-based treatment. Whether the differences in results between these studies might be related to the type of beta blocker used, the patient population studied, the design of the trial, or some other explanation cannot be assessed from the available data. No clinical trial data are as yet available regarding the effects of alpha blockers, angiotensin converting enzyme inhibitors, or calcium antagonists.

The criteria for selection of patients with mild hypertension for drug treatment remain poorly defined. In general, the higher the blood pressure level, the more aggressive should be the drug therapy. In hypertensive patients with diastolic blood pressure below 100 mmHg, and particularly between 90-95 mmHg, opinions differ on when antihypertensive drugs should be instituted. For example, some have advocated, on the basis of the Medical Research Council trial results, that women with mild hypertension should not generally be treated with medications. Others have recommended lowering of blood pressure to below 80 mmHg because of the results of epidemiological studies. Drug treatment appears reasonable, if required to lower blood pressure, in patients with other major cardiovascular risk factors or with evidence of "target organ" damage. However, many important questions remain unanswered regarding the level of blood pressure requiring pharmacologic therapy, the type of medication utilized, the benefits and risks of treatment, and the long-term outcome with respect to cardiovascular complications.

8

ARE SPECIFIC STUDIES IN ELDERLY PATIENTS REQUIRED FOR FDA APPROVABILITY OF A NEW ANTIHYPERTENSIVE DRUG?

W. B. ABRAMS

Merck Sharp & Dohme Research Laboratories,
West Point, Pennsylvania 19486

Response to the question posed in the title of this presentation may be organized into affirmative and negative arguments. Considerations in the affirmative are: (a) Hypertension is prevalent in the elderly, (b) the disorder imparts a substantial risk for mortality and morbidity, (c) there are unique features to the pathophysiology of hypertension in older persons; (d) there are age-associated alterations in organ function and body composition which can alter drug disposition and responses, and (e) specific studies are already being conducted.

Arguments in the negative are none.

PREVALENCE AND RISK

The Joint National Committee on Detection, Evaluation and Treatment of High Blood Pressure defines arterial hypertension as a systolic blood pressure >140 mmHg and/or a diastolic blood pressure >90 mmHg confirmed by two or more readings on two or more visits.(1) Applying this definition, essential hypertension afflicts more than half of Americans older than 65 years of age.(2) Indeed, the National Center for Health Statistics lists hypertensive disease as the second most prevalent disorder in persons aged 65 years and older.(3) Evidence suggests that, left untreated, two-thirds of hypertensive patients in this age group will have heart failure, stroke, heart attack, or dissecting aneurysm within five years.(4,5) Even isolated systolic hypertension, often considered more benign than elevated diastolic pressure, is a major risk factor for cardiovascular and renal disease.(2)

PATHOPHYSIOLOGY

There is some resemblance between the effects of aging and of high blood pressure on the cardiovascular system. When elevated blood pressure is superimposed on changes associated with normal aging, the pathophysiologic result is a state peculiar to older hypertensives.(6)

Elderly <u>normotensive</u> patients exhibit increased vascular stiffness, increased peripheral vascular resistance, cardiac hypertrophy, reduced left ventricular compliance, diminished baroreceptor reflex sensitivity, reduced response to adrenergic stimuli, and a substantial reduction in the glomerular filtration rate and renal blood flow.(7,8) None of these changes are of sufficient degree to be clinically evident or inconsistent with an active life style.

However, when the system is challenged by elevated blood pressure levels, these structural and functional alterations become clinically significant and the patient is exposed to the well-known risks of hypertension, amplified by advanced age.(6) Furthermore, each of these pathophysiologic features of hypertension in the elderly has implications, both positive and negative for drug therapy. The most important qualitative difference between younger and older hypertensives is cardiac output which tends to increase in the former and decline in the latter.(8) Peripheral vascular resistance and blood volume are normal in young hypertensives, but the former is high and the latter is contracted in old patients. The therapeutic goal in elderly hypertensives is to lower peripheral vascular resistance, increase cardiac output, and preserve renal function while at the same time avoiding falls and other risks associated with limited baroreceptor and adrenergic responsiveness.

DRUG DISPOSITION AND RESPONSES

Attainment of this therapeutic goal through drug therapy must take into consideration the age-related changes in body composition, drug elimination mechanisms, and end organ responses which occur in older people.(9) These are listed on Table 1 along with their consequences for drug disposition and responses.

Table 1

Characteristics of the Elderly Relative to Drug Disposition and Responses

1. Reduced renal function: Accumulation of renally cleared drugs
2. Reduced serum albumin and increased alpha-acid glycoprotein levels: Changes in percentage of free drug volume of distribution, and measured levels of bound drugs
3. Relative increase in body fat: Increased distribution volume of fat-soluble drugs
4. Reduction in lean body mass and total body water: Decreased distribution volume of water- soluble drugs

5. Reduction in liver metabolizing capacity: Accumulation of metabolized drugs
6. Decreased cardiac reserve: Potential for heart failure
7. Decreased baroreceptor sensitivity: Tendency to orthostatic hypotension
8. Concurrent illnesses: Disease interactions
9. Multiple drugs: Drug interaction
10. Large interindividual variation: Wide dose range

Item 10 on this list, large interindividual variation, applies to almost all aspects of health care in the elderly. Relative to hypertension, it rules out the construction of treatment recommendations based on age alone. In order to provide guidance for physicians relative to indications, precautions, potential side effects, and dosage of a new antihypertensive agent destined for use in the elderly, specific studies are required.

Fortunately, clinical research practices of the U.S. pharmaceutical industry which evolved from the FDA Discussion Paper of 1983, the FDA/ASCPT Workshop of 1984, and several other symposia around that time provide the experience needed. The practices have been codified as guidelines by Dr. Robert Temple of the FDA and will no doubt be detailed in his presentation to follow.

SUMMARY

In conclusion, there are abundant reasons why specific studies in older patients should be required for approval of new antihypertensive agents and no reasons I can think of why not. In essence, a new drug should be evaluated in the population in which it will be used. This certainly applies to high blood pressure in the elderly.

REFERENCES

1. Joint National Committee. Arch. Intern. Med. 144:1045-1057, 1984.
2. Frohlich, E.D., Gifford, R.W.,Jr., Hall, W.D. J. Am. Coll. Cardiol. 10(suppl A):57A-59A, 1987.
3. Guralnik, J.M., FitzSimmons, S.C. In: Cardiology Clinics (Eds. Abrams, W.B. and Frohlich, E.D.), W. B. Saunders Company, Philadelphia, 1986, pp. 175-183.
4. Svardsudd, K., Tibbin, G. Acta Med. Scand. 205:483-492, 1979.
5. Kannel, W.B., Gordon, T. Bull NY Acad. Med. 54:573-591, 1978.
6. Abrams, W.B. Am. J. Med. 85(suppl 3B):7-13, 1988.
7. Messerli, F.H., Sundgaard-Riise, K., Ventura, H.O., et al. Lancet II:983-986, 1983.
8. Lakatta, E.G. J. Am. Ger. Soc. 37:780-790, 1989.
9. Rocci, M.L.,Jr., Vlasses, P.H., Abrams, W.B. In: Cardiology Clinics (Eds. Abrams, W.B. and Frohlich, E.D.), W. B. Saunders Company, Philadelphia, 1986, pp. 213-225.

9

DO WE NEED ANY MORE ANTIHYPERTENSIVE DRUGS: THE VALIDITY OF A CHANGE IN BLOOD PRESSURE AS THE ONLY ENDPOINT FOR APPROVABILITY

N.M. KAPLAN

Department of Internal Medicine, The University of Texas Southwestern Medical Center, 5323 Harry Hines Boulevard, Dallas, Texas 75235-8852

A change in blood pressure is likely the only practical criterion, along with apparent safety, for approval of a new antihypertensive agent. However, there is a hierarchy of possible and potential endpoints beyond simple antihypertensive efficacy than can be considered as criteria for approvability (Table). Brief consideration will be given to each of these, starting from the bottom and proceeding upward.

Without knowledge of the specific causes of most hypertension, it is now impractical to expect that drugs can be judged on the basis of their ability to reverse specific pathogenetic mechanisms. Nonetheless, knowledge about the effect of individual drugs on various basic defects in both experimental models and hypertensive patients extends beyond the interest of basic pharmacologists. Clinical investigators who perform phase 3 and 4 studies and who write and talk to practitioners about the choice of agents are particularly interested. Their interest arises both from an inherent desire to know the underlying mechanisms by which drugs work to lower the blood pressure and from the hope that knowledge of the effects of individual drugs on these mechanism can provide insight into the relative importance of these mechanisms in the pathogenesis of the hypertensive process.

The next item - prevention of progression - may be almost as difficult to document since the progression of the pressure, its causes, and its consequences are so erratic. In the absence of a marker to identify those who are now normal but destined to proceed into persistent hypertension, it is necessary to wait until the hypertensive process is well established, which may be too late to study the effect of measures that are truly preventative. However, with sufficiently large numbers of subjects who are still free of obvious hypertensive sequelae, it might be possible to examine the effect of a drug versus a placebo upon the rate of progression of various features. A number of relatively small studies have shown at least transient relief of elevated blood pressure and both functional and structural defects after antihypertensive agents have been used and then discontinued. The fragmentary evidence now available suggests that all agents which lower the blood pressure seem to be about equal in their ability to prevent the progression of the process, so this criterion - even if it were practical - might not prove to be any more discriminatory than just the ability to lower the blood pressure.

Protection from target organ damage has been the most actively pursued criterion for proving the benefit of antihypertensive therapy. However, the demonstration of such protection has not been required as a necessary or sufficient criterion for approval of a new drug. In view of the tremendous expense and work required to demonstrate the partial benefit of currently available agents upon target organ damage, it seems unlikely that such evidence can be required for approvability.

On the other hand, the next criterion - reversal of cardiovascular changes, both structural and functional - may be practical at present and even more so in the near future as simpler, less expensive, non-invasive technology becomes available to measure these changes in large populations. For the foreseeable future, this is likely the only possible additional criterion that can be expected to be required for approval.

With recognition of the difficulty in using additional criteria, the final question - Do we need any more antihypertensive drugs? - can be considered. Those now available have obviously been shown to reduce the blood pressure. Limited evidence suggests that their use may reverse cardiovascular changes. Even stronger evidence, from at least 11 large clinical trials, supports their ability to protect against strokes and perhaps renal damage.

Unfortunately, the ability to protect against the target organ damage that is of most importance - coronary ischemia - has not been demonstrable. Moreover, as the search for this evidence has been expanded, a propensity for drug-induced falls in blood pressure to *accelerate* the progression of coronary ischemia has surfaced.

On the basis of what is now known, there does appear to be a definite need for more antihypertensive drugs and for the use of additional criteria of their benefit before they are approved. The costs may seem exorbitant but the need to ensure long-term benefit seems even greater as we continue to expand life-long active drug therapy to the 300 million or more hypertensive patients throughout the world.

Table. ENDPOINTS FOR APPROVABILITY.

Now Possible
Reduction in Blood Pressure
Reversal of Vascular Changes
- Hypertrophy: cardiac, arterial
- Hemodynamics

Protection from Target Organ Damage
- Stroke
- Coronary disease
- Renal damage

Potential
Prevention of Progression
- Blood Pressure
- Hypertrophy
- Hemodynamics

Reversal of Pathogenetic Mechanisms
- Sympathetic nerve overactivity
- Cellular transport defects
- Insulin resistance/hyperinsulinemia

10

THE COST AND TIME TO DEVELOP A NEW ANTIHYPERTENSIVE DRUG DEPENDING UPON THE ENDPOINT

HAROLD K. MARDER, M.D.
GARY LITTMAN, Ph.D.

INTRODUCTION

Pharmaceutical clinical research departments frequently prepare developmental programs for new agents. For any given indication, these plans invariably differ among companies due to unique perspectives and practices within the company; however, most often, the plans follow guidelines for drug development that are issued by the Food and Drug Administration.

The most recent draft guidelines for antihypertensive drug development were released by FDA in May 1988. These guidelines were developed in cooperation with an ad hoc committee of the American Society of Clinical Pharmacology and Therapeutics. They assume that reduction in diastolic blood pressure is a sufficient efficacy endpoint for drug approvability. This presentation will focus on the implementation of those guidelines in the environment of a large, multinational pharmaceutical company. The effects of alternative efficacy endpoints on the time and cost of anti-hypertensive development will be considered.

IDEAL DEVELOPMENTAL PLAN

The proposed clinical pharmacology guidelines for the development of a new antihypertensive agent are summarized in Table 1.

Table 1. Proposed antihypertensive guidelines - clinical pharmacology

- Pharmacokinetics and Metabolism
  - Bioavailability
  - Elimination route and kinetics
  - Food effects
  - Unique demographic characteristics
    - Age
    - Race
    - Disease state
    - Drug interactions
- Pharmacodynamics
  - Mechanism of action
  - Extra-circulatory effects
  - Dose-response
    - Monotherapy
    - Combined with a diuretic
  - Time-effect relationships

The pharmacokinetic requirements are similar to those for other drug classes and do not present any unique developmental or scheduling problems. One or more pharmacodynamic studies should be performed to define the mechanism of action of the antihypertensive in man. It is also necessary to evaluate the important extra-circulatory effects of a new compound. The number and type of these studies are determined by the class of drug under evaluation. For example, a vasodilator would require studies of renal hemodynamics and effects on sodium handling while a beta-blocker would require data about its effects on bronchial smooth muscle.

Careful characterization of dose-response and time-effect relationships has been stressed by the Cardio-Renal Division of FDA. These studies provide the data required to define the most rational dosing of the drug within the approved labelling. These studies comprise a significant portion of the cost and time to develop a new antihypertensive drug.

As appropriate evaluation of dose-response would delineate the "no-effect", minimum effective and maximum effective and/or tolerated doses. This information is frequently obtained in one or more trials of parallel design. A variety of doses, spanning the presumed dose-response curve, and placebo are usually included. Dose-response studies may contain a sufficient number of patients in each assigned dosage limb to detect clinically meaningful differences with statistical significance. Such a well designed trial could serve as one of the two required pivotal efficacy studies.

Dose-response information in the presence of background diuretic therapy is requested for the development of non-diuretic antihypertensives. FDA has introduced the multifactorial study design as one recommended approach to this requirement (Table 2).

Table 2. Multifactorial study design

		DRUG B		
		Placebo	Dose 1	Dose 2
	Placebo			
DRUG A	Dose 1			
	Dose 2			

Placebo and two or more doses of test drug and diuretic are combined in a multicelled study. If appropriate numbers of patients are entered, a trial of this design could provide sufficient dose-response data for approval of both the new single product and an antihypertensive-diuretic combination product.

The importance of the complete delineation of time-effect relationships reflects the emphasis that drug companies have placed on medications that can be administered once daily. To achieve 24 hour coverage, very large single doses have been evaluated in recent registration filings. This approach has produced large declines in blood pressure at the peak of the response and has increased the incidence of both hypotensive and dose-related non-hypotensive adverse drug reactions. Valid peak and trough blood pressure measurements, characterized in an appropriately large population sample, are now an unequivocal requirement for all registration packages. Guidelines clearly specify that trough reductions in diastolic blood pressure should be no less than 1/2 to 2/3 of the peak effect. Dosing regimens need to be evaluated until these criteria are met.

The efficacy and safety requirements for a new antihypertensive are summarized in Table 3.

Table 3. Proposed antihypertensive guidelines - clinical efficacy and safety

Efficacy	
Placebo controlled trials (2)	
Comparison with standard therapy	
Efficacy in special forms of hypertension	
Safety	
Total exposure:	1500
> 2 Weeks:	1000
> 6 Months:	500

The pivotal efficacy studies should be placebo controlled and have a duration of at least 4 weeks. Most of the recent dossiers have contained trials of 8 weeks duration. Additionally, at least one study should be performed against a standard comparator. Unless the new agent is truly novel, the comparator should be chosen from the previously approved antihypertensives of the same class. The study need not demonstrate superiority of the new agent; however, it should be empowered to detect statistical significance if a clinically meaningful efficacy difference exists. This trial should have a minimum duration of 3 months. Finally, some data should be provided about safety and effectiveness in patients with severe hypertension and secondary forms of hypertension.

The size of the registration package is not determined by the efficacy and pharmacology information mentioned above, since these data can be derived with far fewer than 1000 patients. Rather, in order to ensure that uncommon adverse reactions are detected, it is necessary to add patients to the plan so that the total number exposed to at least 2 weeks of the drug approximates 1000. In addition, the program must provide safety data from at least 500 patients treated for a minimum of 6 months. These data may be derived from open studies; however, it is always helpful to have a control group to assess the real significance of adverse reactions. Solutions employed by companies to solve this problem range from a variety of comparative trials to open-label uncontrolled studies. The exact approach that is chosen is often based upon marketing as well as research considerations.

The timing of any project is dependent upon the studies that comprise the critical path, the portion of the program that generally must be completed in sequence, rather than in parallel. Table 4 lists the studies that might comprise the critical path in the development of an anihypertensive agent in a typical CR&D department.

Table 4. Critical path studies
Single dose safety study
Multiple dose safety study
Preliminary dose-ranging and duration of action
Parallel group dose ranging
Positive comparator trial
Multi-cell combination trial
Open label safety

Each of the first 2 safety studies must be completed and analyzed before the succeeding portions of the program can proceed. Preliminary dose-ranging and duration of action data are obtained so that correct doses and dosing intervals are chosen for the larger and costlier pivotal studies. The remaining studies may be completed in an overlapping fashion that is dictated, in large part, by resources. Resource allocation usually has a critical influence on the ability of a company to initiate and conduct many large studies simultaneously. In large companies, projects often compete for resources with other projects of similar promise; and in small companies there rarely exists the depth of personnel to commit truly unlimited resources to a project. It would take at least 4 years, and frequently longer, to develop an uncomplicated antihypertensive using the approach delineated above.

The costs for conducting clinical trials vary from sponsor to sponsor. Estimated costs for the program as discussed are approximately $8.5 million (Table 5).

Table 5. Program costs

Phase I:	420 subjects	$ 2.0 million
Phase II:	450 subjects	$ 2.5 million
Phase III:	920 subjects	$ 4.0 million
		$ 8.5 million

These funds only represent direct clinical grant costs and do not include administrative overhead.

A registration package developed along these lines will provide all of the information required to assure that the new drug effectively lowers diastolic blood pressure. Clear instructions will be available to permit the clinician to choose appropriate doses and dosing intervals to achieve the desired antihypertensive effect. Sufficient safety data will be provided to fully characterize common drug-related adverse effects and to detect the vast majority of effects with a prevalence of at least 1%. In summary, the package will contain all of the information necessary to approve a drug to reduce diastolic blood pressure.

ALTERNATIVE EVIDENCE OF EFFICACY

One may argue that existing data have failed to demonstrate that reducing diastolic blood pressure confers benefit to patients with mild or moderate essential hypertension. If this is accepted, it could be argued that approval to market antihypertensive drugs should require data from studies that utilize either different study populations or alternative endpoints of efficacy (Table 6).

Table 6. New developmental approaches

Different patient populations
Morbidity and mortality trial
Substitute surrogates

The easiest alternative approach to accept, from a theoretical perspective, would probably be a redefinition of the study population. A cooperative study sponsored by the Veteran's Administration and published in 1970 demonstrated that blood pressure control provided protection against the cardiovascular complications induced by hypertension in patients with diastolic blood pressure between 105 and 114 mm Hg. Two placebo controlled clinical trials could, theoretically, be performed in this population. Presumably, one of the trials would have to evaluate multiple doses in a parallel design. The disadvantages of this approach are obvious. First, the rate of patient recruitment would reflect the relative paucity of patients with stable diastolic blood pressure above 104 mm Hg. Second, institutional review boards could raise objections to the use of placebo in these patients for up to 12-16 weeks (including baseline, washout, and trial periods). Even if placebo treatment was acceptable, it would probably require the population to be confined to patients with diastolic blood pressures of less than 114 mm Hg to avoid life-threatening complications of hypertension. Finally, this approach would restrict the indicated use of the drug to the population that was studied. This restriction undoubtedly would prove untenable for commercial interests.

The most straightforward test of the value of antihypertensive therapy for the majority of hypertensive patients would be a morbidity and mortality study in patients with mild and moderate essential hypertension. This trial could use non-fatal myocardial infarctions and fatal CHD-related events as the primary efficacy endpoints. Since no available therapy has been established to have a beneficial effect on these endpoints in this population, it would not be sufficient to conduct a study where one "proves equivalence" to a control agent. Rather, utilizing either placebo or a positive control, a significant advantage for the test drug would have to be demonstrated. Conducting such a trial with placebo rather than an active control would seem preferable since identifying an appropriate control agent is problematic. An agent expected to have a relatively neutral effect on coronary risk (e.g. thiazide) would afford the best chance of demonstrating a significant advantage for the test drug but would increase the likelihood of a positive result being interpreted as the control drug doing harm rather than the test drug doing good.

The United States Pooling Project compiled the results of 5 large studies to determine the frequency of non-fatal myocardial infarctions plus fatal CHD-related events in patients with essential hypertension. Their data suggest an incidence of approximately 120 per 1000 over 8 years. Assuming that the test drug would reduce this incidence by 25% relative to a suitable control, a study that could detect this difference with 80% certainty would require approximately 3500 patients with follow-up for 8 years. Assuming a minimal annual cost of $1500 per patient, a sponsor would risk approxmiately $42 million to test a totally unproven hypothesis.

If such a trial were to be conducted, an added complication would be the development in some patients of "intermediate endpoints" (e.g., persistent proteinuria, azotemia or moderately severe hypertension) that would require drug treatment. Regardless of whether or not placebo were involved in the trial, it would be necessary to provide such patients with standard treatment, either in place or in addition to study drug. One could perform an analysis with these intermediate conditions included among the endpoints; however, for such an analysis to have a primary role, there must be a consensus that preventing anything in the expanded set of endpoints is an acceptable goal. In addition, patients receiving standard treatment could be followed to see whether any of the original endpoints occur. An analysis based on the original endpoints would incorporate the intention-to-treat principle and address the question of whether treatment before the intermediate endpoints develop provides any benefit. While such an analysis would be interesting, it could complicate the overall interpretation of the trial since standard treatment is likely to diminish the differences between groups.

Another approach would be more cost-effective but probably much less persuasive. It would include an analysis of the database to detect effects on a parameter or parameters thought to be important in defining the risk of coronary disease. Left ventricular hypertrophy represents a single parameter that could be quantified with reasonable precision. A more encompassing analysis might include the use of the coronary risk equation derived from the Framingham database and shown in Table 7.

Table 7. Coronary risk coefficients

Variable	Coefficient	
	Men	Women
Age (years)	0.3743307	0.2665693
Age x Age	- 0.0021165	- 0.0012655
Serum Cholesterol (mg/ml)	0.0258102	0.0160593
Systolic Blood Pressure (mm Hg)	0.0156953	0.0144265
Cigarette Smoking *	0.5583013	0.0395348
LVH by ECG *	1.0529656	0.8745090
Glucose Intolerance #	0.6020336	0.6821258
Cholesterol x Age	0.0003619	0.0002157
Intercept	-19.7708560	-16.4598427

* 1 = yes, 0 = no
\# 1 when fasting glucose > 115 mm/ml; otherwise 0

From: Kennel, WB; McGee, D; and Gordon, T.: Am. J. Cardiol. 38:46-51, 1976

Neither of these approaches would add significant cost or time to the program; however, it is obvious that one surrogate, diastolic blood pressure, is merely being replaced by one or more different surrogates. To date, there is no surrogate that has been shown to confer long-term clinical benefit in a prospectively designed study.

CONCLUSION

The current draft guidelines for the development of antihypertensive agents can be met in a program lasting approximately 4 years and costing approximately $8.5 million. An additional 2 to 3 years would be added for the evaluation of the dossier by FDA. If diastolic blood pressure is not accepted as a surrogate of clinical benefit, alternative approaches could involve substitution of similarly problematic alternative surrogates, studies in limited patient populations or performance of a long-term morbidity and mortality trial that would be unrealistic for most sponsors. Such a study would triple the time of drug development and raise the cost by a factor of 5.

Many untested hypotheses are currently accepted as truth by most clinicians. Clearly there is a need to critically evaluate these hypotheses in carefully designed clinical trials. However, one can question the position that requires the pharmaceutical industry to sponsor these evaluations. Seen from one perspective, this task falls within the realm of general medical research rather than drug development research. The pharmaceutical industry has a clear obligation to determine that their drugs are safe and effective; that they produce the effects defined in labeling, that the optimal doses to be used and the adverse effects to be anticipated are well defined. Any advancement in the state of knowledge about the clinical entity being treated should be considered a bonus rather than an absolute requirement for approval.

PANEL ON HYPERTENSIVE TRIAL DESIGN ISSUES

Dr. Moore: Is there any way you can answer the type of subgroup that you are interested in for trial endpoints?

Dr. Temple: Lipids are studied not necessarily in the sophisticated way they would be for lipid lowering agents but you get a reasonable idea and if a company perceives the potential advantage there they will persue it reasonably diligently. LVH is gaining interest as something to study, and I think we will see people doing that. Another possibility is that Dr. Lipicky has recently completed an effort that involved pulling the results of all the anti-anginal trials that we would find that used the placebo to see if anybody was being hurt by being in placebo-controlled trials because people were objecting to them and the results were gratifying. You seem to be doing slightly better if you are not on active drugs as far as morbid events. Such possibilities probably exists in other areas. If you had large numbers of placebo-controlled trials, possibly you could address some of those questions.

Dr. Moore: But you are not going to direct the industry to these questions? If they are not asked to do that then they are not very motivated to do it.

Dr. Temple: Are you referring to lipid companies? They do get lipid profiles as part of the controlled trials. They also look at electrolytes and do usual chemistry monitoring. We have not figured out a way to ask people to find out whether the drug decreases the rate of stroke because it cost 42 million dollars to do that study, so that is true that we have not asked for that kind of study. I think we need to look at LVH as something that ought to be inquired about.

Dr. Kaplan: Part of the problem is that you all don't want to include patients that are the ones that need to be looked at as you develop a new drug. You exclude anybody who's had any kind of overt cardiovascular problem because you don't want someone to die in a drug study. We have a problem that our human research committees will not allow us to study patients who are the ones who need to be studied. Dr. Temple brought up an issue that he doesn't believe in the J curve and the reason that I think we haven't seen it is because the studies have excluded people with pre-existing or known overt cardiovascular disease before they are brought into a study. HDFP did a very careful job of trying to exclude those people. Certainly, any clinical trial involved in developing a new drug is going to exclude those people. So we can't ask you to provide us those data.

Dr. Chobanian: I am depressed about how long it is going to take to get outcome data. If you look at the NIHs budgets and the discussion at committee levels, it looks as if it is going to be almost impossible to mount very large clinical trials on the basis of NIH funding and the industry is not going to do it for the average drug.

It may be an unusual situation when industry does it. I think dollars are an issue. My own feeling would be that in some way, the FDA ought to reduce requirements in terms of some of the accessory things that companies have to do to cut the cost down but then in someway set aside dollars in post-marketing studies that would be used so that the total expenditures might not be a huge amount. From my standpoint I am not as concerned about whether 12-1/2 or 20mg is the right dose, but I am concerned about whether the bigger outcome is going to be different.

Dr. Irvin: I agree with what you are staying about the outcome of endpoint studies. I think a great job was done for a clinical plan for the next new antihypertensive agent. I think one thing that we did not discuss as well as we should is what effects has antihypertensive therapies had over the course of the last several years to reduce coronary artery disease even though we have not been able to definitely and scientifically prove that I think it is very difficult for us to estimate what these event rates are in planning in future mortality-like studies. I would question the 42 million dollar figure that was discussed this afternoon. This may be an underestimate of the cost of doing such trial. I am not so sure that we know how to figure out how to go about that based upon the efficacy that we've seen from presently available agents.

Dr. Marder: I would certainly agree that it is an underestimate, and I was very careful to do that because people who have spoken on this subject in the past have been criticed for inflating the cost. Clearly there is an enormous cost of actually doing the trial to support all the legistical efforts and that wasn't included at all. I think the cost that I estimated on a per patient basis are also very conservative.

Dr. Temple: There are cheaper ways to do trials. These have been mostly carried out in Europe, but a very long-term trial of aspirin as primary prevention has been carried out in this country for a small cost. We are not talking 40 million we are talking about a couple of million tops for a 22,000 patient trial. If you keep the endpoint simple and don't ask too many hard questions, for example, in the treatment of mild hypertension you might just count bodies at the end of the period and not worry too much about how people died. It's not inconceivable that some of these approaches are useful and they should not be dismissed out of hand because they are not necessarily getting sophisticated baseline measurements.

Dr. Moore: The trouble is, and I was one of the doctors, and it was very nice to take a group of 30,000 patients and you knew you were not going to change their medication or any other thing that might change the data. I can't conceive of that being done in the real work with hypertensive patients. I just don't think that that sort of crude endpoint of overall mortality is going to be practical.

Dr. Temple: How many doctors do you think have hypertension from 90 to 105.

Dr. Moore: I don't know, there may be enough. As long as we have an administration that says "read my lips there will be no more taxes" we're not going to ever have an additional amount of money to spend for medical research in this country. Maybe the public is tired of giving us all that money because we have not spent it very well as far as they are concerned. I don't know what the problems are, but clearly there is not going to be enough money for these kinds of studies in the federal medical research budget. I don't think any pharmaceutical company is going to support in a major way a comparative study of their drug against anything else because they may come out second best, and there is no way you can justify that to your stockholders or to anybody else.

Would each of you who represent a major pharmaceutical company with an antihypertensive in the market be willing to put 1/10 of 1 percent of your current sales away for the NIH to take that money and set-up a proper clinical study. Now that is not irrational to ask that to be done.

Dr. Temple: The third party payors have tremendous interest in finding out whether the new extremely expensive drugs are better in which case it is worth it or not better in which case they can save a lot of money.

Dr. Chobanian: The problem is if you don't mount a clinical trial in the next few years you won't know for the next ten years, and for those who are still going to be around 10 years from now are going to be discussing the same kind of information with new data to talk about. I think there is tremendous justification for looking at outcome. The question is how to do it and how to pay for it, but I don't think you should sit back and say we can't do it because the industry does not want to do it, the government does not want to do it.

Dr. Porush: Dr. Kaplan made a comment about eliminating a relatively large group of patients on the basis sof 24-hour blood pressure monitoring. Did you mean that for study purposes as far as the industry is concerned or did you mean that we shouldn't be treating these people? I think it is clear that we don't have sufficient normal data to know what do to with people who's ambulatory blood pressure is 135/85.

Dr. Kaplan: I was talking about drug companies developing or looking at a new drug.

Dr. Porush: I think it may come through for some us that these are people that we shouldn't be concerned about at all. My other question to Dr. Temple is in view of the new analysis of HDFP in regards to kidney disease, are there any guidelines about what do we want to see with regard to kidney function and antihypertensive drugs? I think that whole issue is turning around. Ten years ago, if the drug improved renal blood flow it was a great drug, and now a drug that improves renal blood flow may be a bad drug for the kidney.

Dr. Temple: It hasn't been yet given any thought by me. I was unaware of the analysis that you are describing. We certainly look at short-term effects on renal function as measured in the usual fashion. What was the finding?

Dr. Porush: The study from Birmingham showed that inspite of blood pressure control renal function may deteriorate. There may be a factor related to drugs, and I think the HDFP analysis by Schulman is just an analysis about the importance and significance of renal insufficiency in a group of patients with essential hypertension.

Dr. Temple: The early data showed that one of the benefits that was obtained, probably no single endpoint by itself would have come out significant but there were changes in the right direction showed that renal failure was one of the things that you prevented when you lowered blood pressure at least in people with very high blood pressure. That's one of the markers that it seems to me we want the answer to. We want to know whether the old drugs and the new drugs are different but I don't see how we can do that aside of the contents of a huge study.

Dr. Kaplan: I think there are people in the audience involved in studies certainly in diabetics with early nephropothy who are looking at the effects of these drugs on renal function. I would assume calcium blockers too are being looked at in that regard. I assume that some modest size studies are in the process now to look at these particular class of drugs on renal function.

Dr. Temple: But what those are looking at are people with developed abnormalities and to see whether you can reverse them. That may be a important question. The other question is whether people who are treated successfully with one or the other of these drugs will develop renal dysfunction and that must be a fairly rare event and means large studies.

Dr. Kobelt: I have a question about the dose ranging studies in the development of combination therapy. Dr. Lipicky presented in the morning the factorial design and beside this factorial design he showed the dose escalation study with the Non-Mem analysis. I would like to know if this is an alternative or does he consider this an additional possibility to make dose ranging studies in the combination development.

Dr. Lipicky: I don't think that that has been addressed from the advantage point of the design or the analysis Non-Mem type for looking at combination therapies. There is no theoretical reason that one would think it would not be able to be done. What one would actually have to do has not been thought through to my knowledge by anyone and there is certainly no result that one has to look at yet with respect to whether or not if one did design an appropriate experiment and then use that technique to do an analysis if in fact one would get anything from it. I theory it should work and in theory one ought to be able to get dose reponse information for two drugs at the same time, alone and in combination with fewer patients than would be necessary in a factorial design. The major problem clearly is that the analysis part of that is a model dependent analysis, and within FDA the idea of having model dependent analysis be used to hypothesis test and to get a combination approved clearly one needs to demonstrate that A plus B is better than A or B in some kind of hypothesis testing fashion. That's not so clear.

Dr. Kobelt: But this is also true for the factorial design or isn't it?

Dr. Lipicky: Yes it could be if it turned out that the factorial design found what the statisticians call an interaction term that is either 1 or 0. Doing a standard ANOVA analysis which is one way of analysis the factorial design basically is statistically frowned upon, and consequently our statisticians would be unwilling to apply an ANOVA and then draw inference from whatever numbers came from that analysis and then one would be stuck with doing response surface type analyses to draw inferences and then one is in the model dependent area. Clearly, doing model dependent analysis and attempting to better estimate shapes from the advantage point of making decisions is something that is actively being thought about but it is a departure from a hypothesis testing mode of operation and how successful it will be has yet to be determined.

Dr. Temple: Fortunately, most of these more exotic studies that have potential model dependency also have enough data in them so you can look at them in a more mundane way and get some answers. For example, the factorial design studies so far have had group sizes of 25 to 30 and with that group size you can show a difference between the high dose and the placebo. So you can worry about dose reponse trends and surface analyses to refine the whole study, but you don't have to depend on that analysis for all the evidence that your drug works. Dr. Lipicky has taken the position in the past with respect to approving a combination that getting the dose response relationships with the combinations are nice, but what you really have to have is evidence that the combination of the drugs at their usual doses have a bigger effect than the single drugs at the same dose, that is the traditional combination policy. Also, you can be doing a titration study of drug A, drug B and the combination that is suitable for analysis by Non-Mem and other methods. You can then do a lot more with and try to get dose response information using Non-Mem procedures, but it ought to be possible to satisfy the requirements of the combination policy just by using the comparison as people have always done. I think there are emperical ways to dance through this even while you search the data for more information.

Dr. Kaplan: Most of the data that we have on blood pressure endpoints have come from outside the United States. The two major trials that we did after the VA cooperative study have all been done with the attitude that we now have and that is if you can't do a placebo trial in hypertension (and I know that some of the people who are responsible for the design of both HDFP and MRFIT are here) they designed trials very inadequately to study the issue as to the treatment of mild hypertension. Both HDFP and MRFIT provided therapy to both groups. It was just a matter of more therapy to one group than the other. As a result of that I think the data did not come out nearly as strong as it could of if we would have had a truely non-treated half of the population. I know that that was done because we hear in the United States have made the assumption that any degree of hypertension is evil and you cannot leave people untreated. Where as the Eurpeans, Australians and the others who have done these studies have continued in the early 70s and 80s to leave people untreated. Thus, I think we are going to have to make a change in the way we look at hypertension.

Dr. Metz: It is an interesting idea, but Dr. Kaplan appropriate recognized that if you are looking at a risk to benefit assessment there is a heavy risk for the industry. You have to somehow increase the benefit and if that perhaps was in the form of an increased patent life for the companies that contributed and participated in that kind of program then that might get some attention. Dr. Temple or Dr. Lipicky would you like to comment on that?

Dr. Temple: The bulk of people in the mild hypertensive range are thought to deserve therapy now so that all of the agents that are coming out are being used, but people are asking whether that makes sense. So the benefits of the present patent life are being highly realized. The question is whether the data on when they should be used will become available? Congress deals with patent extension, and they have been persuaded in some special cases where the company has put out a lot of money.

Dr. Lipicky: No one was particularly concerned about using blood pressure lowering for a surrogate for clinical benefit for the approval of the new agent. If it is that well established from the advantage point of lowering blood pressure is a clinical benefit, how important do you rank this business of really needing to know whether a new agent compares in the morbitity and/or mortality sense to the agents that have been used in the past because if it is important enough to sort of enter into negotiations or to be able to be looking for funding sources or something like that I am curious as to why somebody today didn't say "FDA you should not be satisfied with simply letting blood pressure lowering be the surrogate for introducing a new antihypertensive". How do you rationalize wanting to raise funds to do studies to provide vital information but still staying that it is perfectly okay to use the surrogate?

Dr. Kaplan: I don't think it's fair to ask newer drugs that are coming on the market are in the same classes they have already been improved. So if you have a new calcium blocker is the FDA going to require your company to prove that calcium blocker prevents mortality and morbitity whereas the other four calcium blockers are already approved have not had to have that data? I don't that is fair.

Now, if you say from now on that all new drugs accepted are going to have to show that data that is another issue.

<u>Dr. Lipicky:</u> Your argument is that you would like to see morbitity and mortality as a criteria for approval, but do you think that it would not be equitable? There have been so many that have already been approved without that evidence.

<u>Dr. Kaplan:</u> We really do need those data to make the kinds of valid comparisons between the different drugs and to know about more drugs being made available without any particular need for them. I would say that the sort of things that are evolving here and that is to be able to do cheaper studies with multiple drugs that are supported by more than one company is not unfeasible. I haven't really sat down and thought about this before but I think it is something in the realm of reason. But to require a new drug developed by one company to have that endpoint proved before the approval of that drug I don't think that is practical.

<u>Dr. Chobanian:</u> I would think that in the next five years we are not going to see any new drugs coming from different classes probably. So we are stuck with variations on the same theme. We will probably have several members from each group coming up. I don't think for approval sake it would be fair to ask for more than the current standards that are set. I would hope that we would change those standards somewhat to make it cheaper and to ask for post-marketing kinds of studies. I don't mean necessarily having mortality trial, but I could forsee seeing high risk groups being treated with multiple risk factors that would go in with multiple interventions and seeing those kinds of trials designed. To ask the same from companies that already have approved drugs will be a difficult thing to do, but I guess one needs to be imaginative and find out how it can be fair across the board. I don't think that we are going to get very far in terms of answering the questions we've raised today.

<u>Dr. Lipicky:</u> But you could see a trial where one arm was calcium channel blocker, but that arm contained several such agents and another arm would be various ACE inhibitors. If one could be clever enough to figure out how to blind it so that it would be class comparisons to something (ignoring what the

control would be). Is that the kind of information you are thinking about?

Dr. Chobanian: That all depends. I would not want to make that as a generalization. There are certain things you can compare on the basis of class effects and there are others you probably cannot. I think one needs to look at the drug and say which one would be comparable that you could consider it as a class, but there are calcium antagonists for example that are all together different in terms of which receptors they interact with, etc. I don't think I would go that far.

Dr. Lipicky: The only reason I asked that question is that if one isn't saying that each new drug is going to have to do something that is related to morbitity and mortality (either preapproval or postapproval) and then one wants to have some kind of cooperative event then basically one needs to think in terms of not having a particular drug singled out. Otherwise one is saying I want every drug studied. Then the feasibility of such a suggestion needs to have a little more thought.

Dr. Temple: I want to address the question of how you can want data and not insist on it in advance. We have a fair number of priors here and they can't be ingnored most of the large studies have shown that at least diuretics and beta-blockers have a favorable effect on overall morbitity so there is a lot of reason to think that lower blood pressure is a good predictor. But that is not a reason for assuming that they are all going to behave the same.

So it doesn't seem unreasonable to continue to approve drugs that lower blood pressure based on what is really a good amount of data indicating that that is a good thing and still wish to know whether there are distinctions between the drugs that could be discovered if people look.

What about a study of this kind? Suppose you took people who developed left ventricular hypertrophy presumably reflectiong poor control in the past and randomly assigned them to two of the therapy modes that might be different and yet both of which seem reasonably valid things to give to people like that. For example, a beta-blocker, a diuretic arm and a calcium channel blocker might not have to be as large as some of the other studies we've described because those people are relatively high risk. If one added Dr. Lipicky's suggestion of using a whole bunch of different drugs so that the data would be uninterperable or generalizable maybe that is the sort of thing that different companies could agree on.

Dr. Marder: Would you conclude that if ACE inhibitors and calcium channel antagonists beat the beta-blocker/thiazide combination would you conclude that that was a true effect or would you be concerned that there would be a negative effect due to changes in lipids etc. from the alternative regimen?

Dr. Temple: The available placebo controlled data doesn't for the most part suggest an adverse effects of beta-blockers. That needs to be discussed at some length. You want to be sure that you are not making a big expensive mistake. My guess is that it would probably would be reasonably assured that it was not doing harm.

Dr. Kaplan: Just like the secondary trials on coronary disease, you certainly are not asking the companies to compare themselves against somebody else. They were only asked to show that there was protection in that high risk group from recurrent myocardial infarction. They are perfectly able now to go out and say that your drug has shown this kind of protection, therefore, it is indicated for that purpose.

Dr. Temple: It's worth commenting in respect to the study we are talking about that as far as beta-blockers and secondary hypertension goes we have been absolutely drug specific. That has a certain kind of fairness and maybe that is one reason for it. But another is that it seemed too important a queston to make a guess on and if you weren't really sure that the drugs were all the same.

Dr. Calhoun: It seems to be an obvious disagreement in terms of the existence of a J curve. I believe Dr. Temple suggested a trial where he purposely pushed the diastolic blood pressure down to 80. I was wondering if Dr. Kaplan would think that is helpful or not in resolving this issue, if not what else could be done to address this issue specifically?

Dr. Kaplan: I have no problems with anybody doing it I think that they better be careful, and that they better look at the endpoints as they and not assume that it is going to be helpful. If you took a bunch of diabetics then I think it will be a lot better to justify that because there is evidence that very low pressures in them may be protective. But if you are looking at people with pre-existing coronary disease that is identifiable then I think it seems to me there is a significant risk in doing that, therefore, I would not approve that study.

Dr. Calhoun: What do you think the risk is? That they will develop angina?

Dr. Kaplan: Unfortunately, most of them have been sudden deaths.

Dr. Temple: Why should they get that?

Dr. Kaplan: Coronary ischemia setting off arrhythmias.

Dr. Temple: Usually went you don't perfuse you get angina.

Dr. Kaplan: I'm not so sure that angina was not also included. Some studies include both morbitity and mortality, but I would say out of the 7 or so most of them are just mortality.

Dr. Temple: I was wondering about whether there is some funny association whether the people who got the low blood pressures could be pushed that low had problems with cardiac function that weren't recognized. These are not randomized trials. They are observational. It seems to me that an absolutely essential part of the hypothesis if you think poor perfusion is a problem is that they ought to be getting angina.

Dr. Kaplan: I don't recall just morbitity data being indentified in any of these because most of them did use death. I think it was an acute myocardial infarction or death as the two endpoints.

Dr. Irvin: It appears that the majority of the time one is going to have an increase incidence or a reported increase in incidence of adverse events by virtue of design. The question then becomes one of even though that is a result of the design of the trial that you will probably pick up increase adverses, how will that effect labeling or will it effect labeling at all as compared to all of the data you have in the controlled trials that the incidence reported in those will probably be lower?

Dr. Lipicky: I don't think that quality of life is reasonable as a surrogate for morbitity or mortality. It certainly is a clinical benefit. It certainly doesn't hurt to know something about it particularly if one is searching around for clinical benefits that are measurable and that is one. I see no problem with that. It is difficult to know what to do with when one gets it, but it might come in handy if the drug has particularly adverse effects.

Dr. Moore: The one study that has looked at this carefully was the captopril versus propanolol versus methodopa study. Captopril was the least bothersome but the least effective and so one would have to insist on equal levels of blood pressure reduction before one would accept comparative data on quality of life. I think those people on captopril had to take more diuretics and when they took more diuretics to get an equal reduction in blood pressure most of the differences dissapeared between the drugs.

Dr. Lipicky: The answer to the second part of your question is that it depends on how Dr. Temple feels that morning. You frequently encounter different incidences of adverse effects. The nature of the way in which the data were collected and as to whether or not the difference in the incidence of adverse effects is information that would be important with respect to how one would view the drug would determine whether it would get into labeling. I think frequently you see in labeling today a number of different sets of adverse reactions that were obtained under different conditions and it sort of says that this was acquired under this set of conditions, etc. I guess the answer is it would probably appear in labeling if it was reasonable for it to appear there.

Dr. Irvin: But if we are going to use quality of life as an endpoint aren't we going to have some kind of standarized method to be able to study it?

Dr. Temple: No. The whole quality of life discussion has a bizzare quality to me it is as if nobody has thought about side effects before. It is as if people didn't know that people feel tired on beta-blockers or that their mouth is dry on methodopa or that they get sleepy on clonidine. What is the new discovery here? Captopril, which does not have those side effects was less bothersome than methodopa is not the greatest discovery. It is self evident as soon as you look at any of the trials of the drug. It's perfectly good to compare two drugs to see what there side effect profile is. But the ideal of reducing valuable information like you get dry mouth on this one and you get a rash on this into a numerical scale is incomprehensable to me. Why loose information you've gone to collect. So of course you should study the properties of your drug and see if people aren't as fatigued or aren't as impotent etc.

<u>Dr. Moore:</u> Do you think that the rules for demonstrating safety are going to change? Is it fair to approve other drugs under that guideline and then to change the guideline to say that you have to show longer-term safety.

<u>Dr. Temple:</u> You don't gain much by doubling that you have to really go another order of magnitude and I guess we've generally felt that that's under the present conditions difficult. There are mechanisms though, mostly developing in England, that really do allow you to assemble 10,000 patients with not that much effort.

<u>Dr. Lipicky:</u> But those numbers aren't controlled clinical trial numbers either so that from the advantage point of what one is oriented towards is simply having a large enough experiential database that if things are happening at a frequency much above a few percent that probably one has a reasonable probability of recognizing it preapproval and incorporating it into the thought process that leads to the final judgment. The major problem with all of this safety issue is that most of the long-term safety comes from uncontrolled databases and it makes that information very difficult to deal with and makes it very hard to make appropriate value judgments if indeed something unfortunate does happen. But, there isn't any anticipation of changing those rules because again it becomes one of those problems of how to do that.

<u>Dr. Temple:</u> One more thought on the question of whether safety databased could be larger. We all imagine that it's very difficult for a company to get

together another 1,000 patients and any suggestion to that affect would really be troublesome and while we sit there thinking that companies are out there putting 20,000 patients in studies without being asked to by us, I know they are being asked by somebody I guess. They are thinking enough of those studies to include data from them in promotion. Not only that we have seen one case where reasonable good data seemed to have emerge it turned out to be adverse. We always tend to think of Richard Peto of inventing the large simple cheap study but these are not quite as cheap as his but they are large and they are relatively simple and they can assemble huge cohorts in a very short order. It may be that we've dismissed the possibilities of making valid use out of those too quickly because they certainly do assemble large databases fast and they do get reports. It might be possible to learn an order of magnitude more without spending very much.

Dr. Frank: I'd like to get back to what is required for FDA approvability. I would like to refer to peak trough. I'm wondering if were are going overboard with the strict definition of a peak-trough ratio. I think you are measuring efficacy at peak and you are not seeing undue reductions in blood pressure. Is there a need for a specific ratio?

Let me give an example, say you do three dose levels of a drug placebo controlled study and your trough measures come out 4,6 and 8 at trough at a dose response and at peak they are 10, 12 and 14 the same. If you take a top dose, 6 to 14 you are about 60 percent, so your diastolic blood pressure has met efficacy. The middle dose 6 versus 12 again the trough measure is at 50 percent, at the botton end with a 4mm reduction your actually meeting the guidelines of greater than 3mm it would be efficacious at trough yet 4 versus 10 you are going to be 40 percent. So if you use a strict ratio you could come around with the suggestion that a lower dose is efficacious as a starting dose and yet it wouldn't meet the criteria from a peak trough yet its peak effect is not excessive it is not a safety worry. Why are we locking ourselves into a stricter ratio.

Dr. Lipicky: The data that you have described would be acceptable.

Dr. Temple: The labeling might say that at the low dose the effect disapears at 24-hours.

Dr. Frank: My question is that you are still locking yourself into a ratio.

Dr. Lipicky: It is not true. There is no ratio. The percentage that was dreamed up in response to someone asking what can it be so you got an answer.

Dr. Kobelt: I would like to know if the FDA would accept that peak-trough ratio measured by 24-hour blood pressure monitoring.

Dr. Lipicky: Sure, absolutely. Any peak-trough estimate is difficult. I think it is necessary to get some kind of information with the respect to time course. If one has 24-hour monitoring and has some means of being able to pick the drug effect out of that data then basically one has nice clean curve where estimate of peak to trough can be made with reasonable precision. The trick obviously is to pull the drug signal out of all of the things that are goint up and down. If one can manage to do that one has a very nice signal and it is very easy to say here is where it is the biggest that's the peak and here it is before the next dose.

Dr. Temple: One would have to be quite sure. A lot of these trials use a baseline that is time distant from the measurement as patients baseline are used as the control period. If there is a downward drift in any of these studies, that means it is very hard to get actual drug effect.

Dr. Pierce: It was suggested that Dr. Marder as one additional possible endpoint for approvability of antihypertensive beyond blood pressure the use of a derived coronary risk analysis score and I would like to present a theoretical question. If we had a new antihypertensive agent of a completely new class and it has some potentially adverse effect on LDL cholesterol was of such a magnitude that we could project that despite the favorable effect on hypertension that coronary events might be projected to be increased. How would we deal with that in the cardio-renal division? Further if that drug had been tested against another agent and we had looked at LVH and it regressed with this agent, how might that then nulify our potential concerns.

Dr. Kaplan: If it were the twelveth beta-blocker I would disapprove it, but if it were the second of a new class of drugs I would implicate that this is a potential hazard of the use of this drug.

Dr. Temple: Certainly a major adverse effect on cholesterol would be taken very seriously and I guess I would want to know that this has some property that makes it seem worth the risk that it worked when other drugs failed if that is even plausable.

Dr. Lipicky: I am not sure off the top that I would accept some combined risk factor score as being the thing that would trigger that panic.

Dr. Shand: It seems to me as I listen today that we are really into the question of certainty, and that the very large trials that are being thought of to be done is it perhaps time for us to lay a little statistics aside and be only 90% certain that we were doing some good in some of these areas? I think you are into very large efforts, I would very comfortable with just a trend because what you are really trying to find out is whether it will go the other way.

I think a statistician who doesn't accept a model based on the law of that mass action will accept a model for analysis of variance needs to be straightened out.

Dr. Lipicky: I think you are right.

Dr. Temple: Trends seem to be important in cholesterol lowering.

Dr. Lipicky: That is an interesting question, and I guess my translation of your question is if you can't find the funding to do a study that will really answer a question, if you ask the question a little differently and were satisfied with a little less certainty in your answer maybe you could find the funding because you are asking for fewer dollars and I don't think that is a crazy question. Would you be satisfied with knowing that ACE inhibitors don't make things significantly worse than did diuretics etc. My answer is yes that would help. The question is whether that would really significantly change the cost. I don't know the answer to that you would have to look at what power, what beta etc. and see if that would influence the cost.

Dr. Temple: We have a funny view of what things cost. Even if you think the relevant studies would cost 300 million that is less than one year's worth of the money that is waisted on treating people between 90 and 105mmHg. It's odd that we only think of the cost and can't manage to get important questions studied. We are going to use databases to try and answer the questions. It is going to be cheap but probably won't be persuasive.

Dr. Kaplan: It is obvious that you all are making the 300 million dollars so you surely don't want to stop that. Nobody is going to argue that a drug company must spend that money to show that it can't sell its product.

III. SURROGATE ENDPOINTS TO DEFINE RISK VS. BENEFITS

11

WHAT SHOULD BE REQUIRED FOR FDA APPROVABILITY OF A NEW ANTIHYPERTENSIVE DRUG? WHAT IS THE FDA'S VIEWPOINT?

R. TEMPLE, M.D.

Food and Drug Administration, Center for Drug Evaluation and Research, Office of Drug Evaluation I, 5600 Fishers Lane, Rockville, Maryland

I will try not to repeat what has been said earlier. The current guidelines and current policy on what is needed to market an antihypertensive drug are fairly clear. Antihypertensive drugs are approved on the basis of a demonstrated ability to lower blood pressure to a reasonable degree and a reasonably complete characterization of a drug's pharmacokinetic and pharmacodynamic properties, with particular emphasis on dose-response and on patient characteristics that can alter this response. We have not, up to now, sought evidence of diminished end-organ damage or mortality for each new agent, relying instead on the past studies that showed such benefits of lowering blood pressure.

We are interested in such pharmacokinetic features as evidence of non-linear kinetics, presence of active metabolites, the effects of patient characteristics such as age, renal status, and hepatic status, potential drug-drug interactions, and possible pharmacogenetic differences. These pharmacokinetic factors are a major cause of person-to-person variability in response.

We also want to know the pharmacodynamic properties of the agent, including the basic mechanism (e.g., beta-blockade or ACE inhibition), the antihypertensive and other hemodynamic effects, and other effects, including adverse effects, and the relation of all of these properties to dose and plasma concentration. If possible, we want both population mean dose-responses and an idea of individual dose-response. Historically, because dose-response information was not carefully pursued, we have tended to overdose with antihypertensive drugs, and the level of overdose has sometimes been enormous. If 12 1/2 of hydrochlorothiazide is an effective dose, past recommendations of 100-200 may have had important adverse consequences. Most of the adverse metabolic effects of diuretics, glucose intolerance, increased cholesterol, and hypokalemia, etc., are dose related. At very low doses they might not exist at all; at high doses they may affect survival.

The evaluation of an antihypertensive agent should characterize the time course of the antihypertensive effect, both within the day, by peak and trough measurements, and over weeks. In general trough effect should be a substantial fraction of peak effect. It is not reasonable to stretch the dose-interval to the point where effectiveness over the whole dosing interval is not maintained.

There is interest in special subgroup effects, e.g., different responses related to age or race or to other patient characteristics.

The kinds of data needed to show effectiveness have been described. There need to be two well-controlled studies of at least 4 weeks duration showing superiority to a control agent. In a dose-response study evidence of dose response alone might be considered acceptable even if no single two group comparison was significant (in a reasonable size study that is not too likely to happen). If the magnitude of the effect were very small, the drug might not be approvable; in recent years, however, effects of 3-4 mmHg have been accepted because standard comparison therapies yielded the same size effect. The reasons for these smaller effects are not clear. There should also be an adequate sized 3 month comparison with active drug, generally one of the same pharmacologic class. In these studies systolic pressure should not be ignored, even if diastolic pressure is the primary end point. Patients studied should be representative of the general population with hypertension with respect to age, sex, race, and severity of hypertension.

Safety is evaluated in the usual fashion, with adequate total-exposure of a broad population, generally including at least 1500 patients, 1000 for at least 2 weeks and 500 for 6 months. There are a number of possible properties of antihypertensive drugs that need to be screened for, including the ability to cause postural hypotension, as first dose effect, edema, weight gain, heart rate changes, inotropic effects, central nervous system depression, electrolyte effects, ECG effects, especially conduction defects and QT prolongation, alteration of serum lipids, alteration of serum glucose, or changes in renal function. Many effects of interest need special attention. You have to take particular care, for example, to discover sexual dysfunction; it does not come out in ordinary trials unless you look for it. For any drug with CNS activity, it may be useful to look specifically for cognitive effects in the elderly. Most antihypertensive drugs should have a careful examination for the possibility of withdrawal effects.

There are a number of kinds of information that are not requested by the guideline but that are of possible interest. There is no specific requirement for examining the difference between high and low renin states, although this is a potentially important distinction. We do tend to look for differences between blacks and whites, which may be a substitute, although not a precise one, for renin status. We have not asked for evidence that a drug can decrease cardiac hypertrophy, or for any other evidence that the drug can decrease end-organ damage. The possibility of using LVH as an end point is interesting because it can be studied, and because it is of growing interest. Recent reports indicate that relatively small, relatively short studies can show changes in LVH and perhaps distinguish between the effects of different therapies.

A problem, of course, is that it is not clear what we would do with such information if we had it, because the ultimate importance (e.g., effect on survival) of effects on LVH is not well established and we would generally not have information about other critical end points, such as stroke, with the same drugs. One would not want to suggest that an effect on LVH was a major advantage for one agent when it might not be as valuable in other ways. With respect to other possible end points of interest it seems impossible to expect that a single drug company could carry out comparative stroke studies, which would need to be enormous, and one can't very well ask for evidence that coronary disease is improved by treatment because no treatment has yet shown convincing improvement.

The possibility of studying drugs in more severe hypertensives, raised by Dr. Morganroth, is of interest, but if the study is intended to find out whether the drug has the property of lowering blood pressure in that population, there probably is not too much to learn. So far nobody has found a drug that only works in one level of blood pressure. This is a new perception; in the past antihypertensive drugs were labeled according to the exact groups of patients that had been studied, mild, moderate and severe. We do not do that anymore; we just label them for hypertension and try to get a reasonably broad sample of patients in the trials. The basis for the change is that all drugs seem to work in all levels of hypertension; you just may need more than one drug to get more severe elevations down to normal levels. On the other hand, there is clearly a potential difference in the side effects that would be seen with different levels of hypertension and response. Minoxidil, e.g., seems far more likely to cause severe fluid retention in severely hypertensive patients, perhaps because their very large BP response provokes very large "compensatory" responses by the body. It therefore is important to include severe hypertension in the population studied.

It is worth remembering, as we think of why we treat hypertension, just how dramatic the results in the moderate to high pressure group in the Freis study were; this was the group with diastolics of 115 to 129 mmHg. In 70 patients who were given placebo over about 16 months, there were two dissections, a ruptured aortic aneurysm, three renal failures, two acute MIs, two heart failures, four strokes/TIAs and one sudden death. That is, 15 out of 70 patients during a short period had overt disasters. Twelve more patients had either unacceptably increased blood pressure (to at least 130 mmHg diastolic) or had severe funduscopic findings. We just do not see that sort of devastation in trials anymore, and no one can really study it properly because patients cannot be left untreated. What we could conceivably study now is whether we can reduce the much lower frequency of strokes in milder hypertensives and improve cardiovascular mortality. Such studies must be very large and prolonged because the event rates are low.

As you can tell, I think it is still reasonable for antihypertensive drugs to be approved on the basis of evidence that they lower blood pressure. Nonetheless, there are still some major questions that ought to be answered. While they need to be answered I do not think that we can expect a single drug company to address them. They are "larger" questions that will need national scale efforts to answer them; organizations with potential interest in doing so would certainly include NIH, the VA and the drug industry. Third party payers also have a major interest in the answers.

Let me indicate the questions that need to be answered. The first question is how do the newer drugs, the calcium channel blockers, and ACE inhibitors, compare to the older drugs? Most of our data on the benefits of treatment of hypertension comes from studies of thiazides, reserpine, and beta-blockers, all drugs with effects that are well-maintained over the dose-interval. It is not unreasonable to assume that other drugs will have similar effects, but it is not self evident either, and it is a very important question. There is a rush to the new agents (ACE inhibitors, calcium channel blockers) based on their perceived better tolerability and on a variety of other possibly advantageous pharmacologic properties, but that is not the same as <u>knowing</u> they are better or even as good. It seems quite possible, for example, that beta-blockers, known to decrease mortality and recurrent infarction in post-infarction patients, will prove to be similarly beneficial in hypertensives with coronary artery disease, a benefit that calcium channel blockers may lack. Certainly, that could be important in the outcome of treating hypertension.

Comparisons aside, a major question is whether any regimen can be shown to improve cardiovascular mortality. There are a number of possible explanations for why we have so far not been able to show this. One is that we are somehow wrong that there really is not a relationship, or not a major relationship, of hypertension itself to coronary artery disease. Another explanation, one that allows for potential improvement, is that the drugs we have been using have adverse cardiovascular risk effects large enough to override the modest benefit of lowering blood pressure; such adverse effects as decreased glucose tolerance, increased cholesterol, and decreased potassium are the candidate villains. It is worth noting that some of those effects could result from the excessive doses we have been using. If you do not use too much thiazide you do not get much effect on potassium, cholesterol or glucose. Another possible reason for the lack of effect on cardiac mortality is that the major drugs used do not have important effects on LVH. Some newer drugs may not have the metabolic problems previous drugs have had and they may affect LVH more. It is worth noting that some of these questions may be very hard to answer because we are talking about primary prevention of coronary artery disease. No primary prevention treatment has ever showed decreased coronary mortality in a controlled trial even when the studies were fairly large. The largest primary prevention study is the Physicians Health Study, which had to abandon its search for a mortality effect of aspirin and settle for reduced rates of myocardial infarction. Studies of cholesterol lowering agents, in primary or secondary prevention settings also have not generally showed effects on mortality, although some overviews of secondary prevention give encouraging results. So it is a very tall order for any drug to show decreased cardiovascular mortality. Perhaps an effect on the sum of fatal and non-fatal coronary events would be a realistic goal.

Another question that needs to be answered, certainly one that is on the table, is whether drugs differ in their ability to reverse left ventricular hypertrophy, and if so, to what degree it matters.

What all this suggests to me is that there are four major kinds of trials that ought to be done. They are all very tall orders.

The first, and probably the most important, before we spend many billions of dollars on a group of drugs that have not been the subject of mortality or morbidity studies, is to compare the older regimens with the newer ones. One possible way to do that would be, because I think you need more than one drug in each treatment arm, to compare a treatment approach that used diuretics and then beta-blockers as one arm with a regimen that used ACE inhibitors and calcium channel blockers as the other arm. One might also consider a central alpha agonist as another treatment arm. Studies will need to be very large to be able to show differences in stroke prevention, if they exist, differences in effects on renal failure (most antihypertensive drugs will probably be good for this) and to have a chance of seeing differences in cardiovascular mortality and morbidity. A subset of patients could be examined for effects on LVH.

The second major issue, discussed earlier today, is whether the size of the target fall in blood pressure makes any difference. E.g., one might compare a group whose diastolic blood pressure is lowered all the way to 80 mmHg with a group lowered only to 95 mmHg. I am troubled by some of the non-randomized data that is being used to say that somewhat excessive blood pressure falls are dangerous. The recent report of Alderman is worth looking at very closely. This is not a controlled trial, but an analysis of an observational database. It was reported that patients who had a small fall of blood pressure, up to 6 mmHg diastolic and patients who had a large fall of more than 17 mmHg had a 3- to 4-fold excess of heart attacks compared to people who were in the "right" zone, a fall of 7 to 17 mmHg from baseline. I must say that I find this outcome hard to believe. Controlled trials to date have usually been unable to detect any difference between placebo-treated and treated patients with respect to coronary events, and here is found a 3-fold difference between patients with 0-6 mmHg and 7-17 mmHg changes. If such differences exist they ought to be sitting very prominently in such studies as the HDFP and it is hard to imagine that such a large difference could have been missed. Before such analyses come to be accepted as true, it is crucial to subject the question to a controlled trial.

The third major issue that needs to be addressed is whether it makes sense to spend the billions of dollars, and cause the considerable inconvenience, resulting from treating patients in the 95 to 105 mmHg range. It is obviously difficult to show benefit in that population but that does not mean that we should not keep trying.

The last area to consider, but I am not not sure how to get at it, is whether it is the maximum blood pressure effect or the "area under the curve" of the effect that is most important. There are therapies that can produce very smooth day-long responses and these could be contrasted with drugs that allow pressures to fluctuate more during the day.

I hope people interested in hypertension, outcome analyses, and patient care in general will urge the various people in the world who have some money to spend to consider spending some of it on these questions.

12

ARE THERE VALID SURROGATE ENDPOINTS FOR MORTALITY THAT CAN BE USED TO EVALUATE THE EFFECTS OF ANTIARRHYTHMIC DRUG THERAPY?

J. THOMAS BIGGER JR., M.D.

Department of Medicine, Columbia University, New York, New York
and the Arrhythmia Control Unit, Columbia-Presbyterian Medical Center
630 West 168th Street, New York, New York 10032

HOLTER AND ELECTROPHYSIOLOGIC ENDPOINTS

A beneficial effect or an adverse effect of drug therapy on death is difficult to assess in patients with cardiovascular diseases because the death rate is moderate (<10% per year) in most patient groups that are the target of treatment assessment. Since the death rate is modest, studies must be large, long-lasting, and expensive if they are to establish either benefit or harm of a drug in terms of mortality. The realization that the answer to questions about a drug's effect on mortality will be slow in coming and expensive to get naturally raises the issue of surrogate endpoints that may provide reasonable predictions of mortality effects at less effort and cost than full-scale controlled, randomized clinical trials with mortality as an end point. This discussion will focus on the question: what surrogate endpoints are valid and sufficient to establish benefit of an antiarrhythmic drug on mortality.

First, it is worth clarifying the difference between a risk predictor and an indicator of efficacy or harm. Cardiovascular risk predictors have been studied most extensively in coronary heart disease, especially after myocardial infarction. Pulmonary rales occurring in the CCU phase of myocardial infarction, left ventricular ejection fraction, exercise tolerance, ventricular arrhythmias in a 24-hour continuous ECG, late potentials in the signal averaged ECG, low heart rate or heart period variability all have the ability to predict mortality after myocardial infarction (1-8). Patients who have abnormal values of significant magnitude for any of these variables have much higher death rates than those with normal or near normal values. However, not all of these variables can be used as indicators of drug efficacy or harm. For example, we would not expect the response of rales, left ventricular ejection fraction, or late potentials in the signal averaged ECG to drugs to indicate a long-term beneficial effect of antiarrhythmic treatment on mortality (9).

Over the past 10 years, two methods of assessment have been the mainstays for predicting antiarrhythmic drug efficacy and, to a lesser extent, proarrhythmic toxicity. (1) Holter techniques, usually 24-hour continuous ECG recording (with or without exercise testing) and (2) electrophysiologic methods (10,11). We will briefly assess whether surrogate end points derived from either of these methods are valid and sufficient for establishing the mortality effects of antiarrhythmic drugs.

24-Hour Continuous Electrocardiographic Recordings.

Ten years ago, suppression of ventricular arrhythmias was the yardstick by which antiarrhythmic drug efficacy was evaluated. Longitudinal, observational studies established beyond doubt that ventricular arrhythmias predicted a poor outcome (i.e., increased mortality rate) after myocardial infarction independent of left ventricular ejection fraction (12-17). In smaller studies done in patients with congestive heart failure, ventricular arrhythmias were shown to have similar predictive power (18,19). Uncontrolled studies suggested that suppression of spontaneous ventricular arrhythmias was associated with an improved chance of survival (20,21). That is, patients who had either unsustained or sustained ventricular arrhythmias as their clinical arrhythmia and frequent ventricular premature complexes and unsustained ventricular tachycardia in their drug-free Holter recording and whose ventricular arrhythmias were markedly suppressed by antiarrhythmic drugs had a better survival experience than those whose ventricular arrhythmias could not be suppressed during a series of antiarrhythmic drug trials. In these studies, about three-fourths of the patients had their spontaneous ventricular arrhythmias suppressed. In these studies, exercise also was used in the evaluation of efficacy and safety (10,11). There were no patients with recent myocardial infarction in these studies. The Cardiac Arrhythmia Pilot Study (CAPS) showed that three drugs; encainide, flecainide, and moricizine were capable of suppressing ventricular arrhythmias after myocardial infarction and maintaining suppression for one year in most patients (22). The Cardiac Arrhythmia Suppression Trial (CAST) used the same three drugs to test the hypothesis that suppressing ventricular arrhythmias would increase survival rates after myocardial infarction (23).

In April 1989, encainide and flecainide were removed from CAST because it had become very unlikely that they would produce benefit (24). On the contrary, there was strong evidence that encainide and flecainide were increasing mortality after myocardial infarction. From the perspective of our discussion of surrogate Holter endpoints, CAST provides some interesting data. The only patients who were randomized to the main study of CAST were those who had their ventricular arrhythmias suppressed, i.e., 80% reduction of ventricular premature complexes frequency, 90% reduction in episodes of unsustained ventricular tachycardia (3-15 consecutive complexes), and 100% suppression of ventricular tachycardia ≥15 complexes. From CAPS we learned that 70% patients who show this degree of suppression remain consistently suppressed over the course of one year of follow-up (22). Despite this marked degree of suppression, CAST patients treated with encainide and flecainide had an **increased** mortality rate over 300 days of follow-up (24). The difference in mortality rates between the placebo and active treatment groups continued to widen over the 300 days of follow-up. CAST preliminary data showed that the risk ratio for arrhythmic death or cardiac arrest (3.6) was greater than the risk ratios for cardiac death or cardiac arrest (2.5) or non-cardiac death (1.3). These data suggest that the deaths occurring in the encainide/flecainide treated groups during follow-up have an arrhythmic mechanism. Thus, we have a paradox: the indicator of antiarrhythmic drug efficacy predicted a beneficial response while the outcome showed clearcut harm. Clearly, then, the spontaneous ventricular arrhythmias in a Holter recording are not a valid surrogate for mortality. The characteristic of being suppressible by encainide or flecainide is associated with a reduced mortality rate during follow-up even though treatment with these drugs is discontinued at the end of titration. It is possible that ventricular premature complexes are never suitable surrogates for mortality. Although the spontaneous ventricular arrhythmias detected and quantified in 24-hour Holter recordings do predict increased mortality risk, suppression of the ventricular arrhythmias may not predict improved survival. An alternate explanation for the dissociation could be a toxic drug action that overhelms the benefit of suppression. The CAST findings may be drug specific, i.e., the dissociation between suppression and good outcome may be drug specific to drugs with class IC antiarrhythmic action. It remains to be seen whether suppression of spontaneous ventricular arrhythmias will serve as a valid surrogate for mortality for drugs with any class of antiarrhythmic action.

Electrophysiologic Studies as Surrogates for Mortality

Suppression of inducible sustained ventricular tachycardia has been used as a surrogate endpoint indicating improved survival (10-12). Patients who are inducible when drug free and

EVALUATION OF EPS AS A SURROGATE FOR DEATH

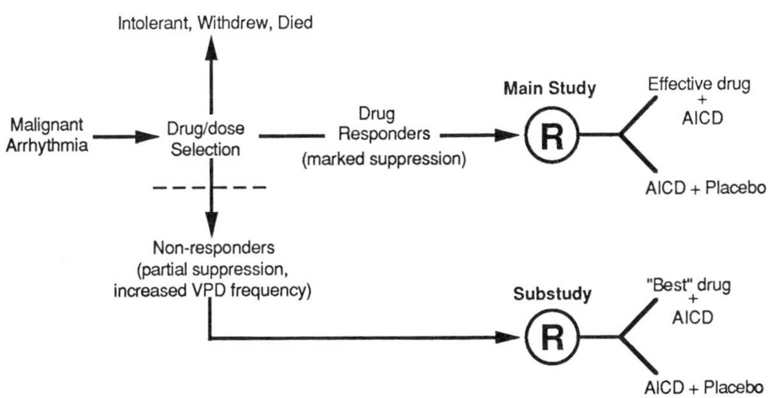

become uninducible during drug treatment are viewed as having their risk substantially reduced as a result of drug treatment. About half of the patients will have this response to one of a series of drugs evaluated. Conversations with FDA officials suggest that this electrophysiologic endpoint is viewed as a valid and sufficient surrogate for mortality. However, the evidence on which this view is based is scientifically weak. The characteristic of becoming uninducible during programmed ventricular stimulation during drug treatment could be associated with a good outcome that does not require continued drug treatment. Since this was the case for encainide and flecainide in CAST, this hypothesis becomes quite plausible for electrophysiologic assessment as well. There has not been a placebo controlled study of the electrophysiologically guided treatment. Therefore, we really do not know which, if any, of the drugs are capable of improving survival. It may be that the patients who are drug responsive would do better if they were taken off their antiarrhythmic drug when serial testing was completed. The reason that such studies have not been done is the ethical concern that effective therapy will be denied patients in the placebo group. However, it would now be possible to test the hypothesis that drug responsiveness is a predictor of good outcome during follow-up that does not require continued use of drug treatment with no risk to the patients assigned to the placebo group. Since treatment of patients with malignant arrhythmias with the automatic implantable cardioverter defibrillator (AICD) yields better results than drugs predicted to be effective by electrophysiologic studies, the design shown in Figure 1 could be implemented ethically.

Conclusion

At the present time, there are no established endpoints that can be considered valid and sufficient surrogates for mortality. Not that there may not be any, but none have been demonstrated. After the preliminary CAST findings, it would seem unwise to accept unproven surrogate endpoints no matter how reasonable they may appear to be.

If there are no valid surrogates for mortality, we must conduct sizable mortality trials to establish the safety of antiarrhythmic drugs. How to conduct adequate mortality trials efficiently and at reasonable cost will be a challenge we must meet in the future.

REFERENCES

1. The Multicenter Post Infarction Research Group. Risk stratification and survival after myocardial infarction. N. Engl. J. Med. 309:331-336, 1983.

2. Greenberg, H., McMaster P., Dwyer, E.M., Jr. and the Multicenter Post-Infarction Research Group. Left ventricular dysfunction after myocardial infarction: results of a prospective multicenter study. J. Am. Coll. Cardiol. 4:867-874, 1984.

3. Dwyer, E.M., Jr., McMaster, P., Greenberg, H.M. and the Multicenter Postinfarction Research Group. Non-fatal cardiac events and recurrent infarction in the year following acute myocardial infarction. J. Am. Coll. Cardiol. 4:695-702, 1984.

4. Krone, R.J., Gillespie, J.A., Weld, F.M., Miller, J.P., Moss, A.J. and the Multicenter Postinfarction Research Group. Low-level exercise testing after myocardial infarction: usefulness in enhancing clinical risk stratification. Circulation 71:80-89, 1985.

5. Bigger, J.T., Jr., Fleiss, J.L., Kleiger, R., Miller, J.P., Rolnitzky, L.M. and The Multicenter Post-Infarction Research Group: The relationships among ventricular arrhythmias, left ventricular dysfunction and mortality in the 2 years after myocardial infarction. Circulation 69:250-258, 1984.

6. Bigger, J.T., Jr. and Steinberg, J.S.: Risk stratification for arrhythmic death after myocardial infarction. In *Cardiac Pacing and Electrophysiology,* El-Sherif, N. and Samet, P., editor, W.B. Saunders Company., Philadelphia, 1989, in press.

7. Kleiger, R.E., Miller, J.P., Bigger, J.T., Jr., Moss, A.J., and The Multicenter Post-Infarction Research Group: Decreased heart rate variability and its association with increased mortality after acute myocardial infarction. Am. J. Cardiol. 59:256-262, 1987.

8. Marcus, F.I., Cobb L.A., Edwards, J.E., Kuller, L., Moss, A.J., Bigger, J.T., Jr., Fleiss, J.L., Rolnitzky, L.M., Serokman R., and the Multicenter Postinfarction Research Group: Mechanism of death and prevalence of myocardial ischemic symptoms in the terminal event after acute myocardial infarction. Am. J. Cardiol. 61:8-15, 1988.

9. Steinberg, D.S., Freedman, R.A, Bigger, J.T., Jr., for the ESVEM investigators: Antiarrhythmic drug therapy and the signal averaged electrocardiogram. In *The Prevention of Sudden Cardiac Death,* El-Sherif, N., editor, New York, 1989, in press.

10. Bigger JT Jr. Long-term continuous electrocardiographic recordings and electrophysiologic testing to select patients with ventricular arrhythmias for drug trials and to determine antiarrhythmic drug efficacy. Am J Cardiol 58:58c-65c, 1986.

11. Bigger, J.T., Jr.: Holter/exercise and electrophysiologic methods for evaluating drug therapy for malignant ventricular arrhythmias: do we need both models? In *Cardiac Arrhythmias: New Therapeutic Drugs and Devices,* Morganroth, J. and Moore, E.N., editors, Martinus Nijhoff, Boston, 1985, 210-221.

12. Bigger, J.T., Jr., Rolnitzky, L.M., Merab, J.: Epidemiology of ventricular arrhythmias and clinical trials with antiarrhythmic drugs. Chapter 59 in *The Heart and Cardiovascular System, Scientific Foundations,* Fozzard, H.A., Haber, E., Jennings, R.B., Katz, A.M., and Morgan, H.E., eds., Raven Press, New York, 1986, 1405-1449.

13. Ruberman W, Weinblatt E, Goldberg JD, Frank CW, Shapiro S. Ventricular premature

beats and mortality after myocardial infarction. N Eng J Med 1977; 297:750-7.

14. Moss AJ, Davis HT, DeCamilla J, Bayer LW. Ventricular ectopic beats and their relation to sudden and nonsudden cardiac death after myocardial infarction. Circulation 1979; 60:998-1003.

15. Mukherji J, Rude RE, Poole KE, et al. Risk factors for sudden death after acute myocardial infarction: two-year follow-up. Am J Cardiol 1984; 54:31-6.

16. Nicod P, Gilpin E, Dittrich H, Henning H, Ross J Jr. Prognostic significance of complex ventricular arrhythmia for cardiac death during the first year after myocardial infarction. J Electrophysiol 1987: 1:93-102.

17. Coromilas J, Bigger JT Jr, Kleiger RE, Rolnitzky LM, Fleiss JL, and the MDPIT Research Group. Relations among left ventricular dysfunction, ventricular arrhythmias, and mortality after myocardial infarction Circulation 80(Suppl II): 48, 1989.

18. Bigger JT Jr. Why patients with congestive heart failure die: arrhythmias and sudden cardiac death. Circulation 75(suppl IV):28-35, 1987.

19. Bigger, J.T., Jr.: How to study sudden cardiac death as an endpoint in congestive heart failure trials. In *Congestive Heart Failure,* Morganroth, J. and Moore, E.N., editors, Martinus Nijhoff, Boston, 1987, 255-262.

20. Graboys TB, Lown B, Podrid PJ, DeSilva R. Long term survival of patients with ventricular arrhythmia treated with arrhythmic drugs. Am J Cardiol 1982; 50:437-443.

21. Lampert S, Lown B, Graboys TB, Podrid PJ, Blatt CM. Determinants of survival in patients with malignant ventricular arrhythmia associated with coronary artery disease. Am J Cardiol 1988; 61:791-797.

22. The Cardiac Arrhythmia Pilot Study (CAPS) Investigators. Effects of encainide, flecainide, imipramine and moricizine on ventricular arrhythmias during the year after acute myocardial infarction. Am J Cardiol 1988; 61:501-9.

23. Bigger, J.T., Jr.: Methodology for clinical trials with antiarrhythmic drugs to prevent cardiac death: US experience. Cardiology 74(suppl II):40-56, 1987.

24. The Cardiac Arrhythmia Suppression Trial (CAST) Investigators. Preliminary Report: Effect of encainide and flecainide on mortality in a randomized trial of arrhythmia suppression after myocardial infarction. N Engl J Med 1989; 321:406-12.

PANEL ON SURROGATE ENDPOINTS: ANTIARRHYTHMIC AGENTS

Dr. Kowey: I think that Dr. Bigger's point about the surrogate for mortality in EP testing is well taken and that really is not a hypothesis which has been adequately tested. However, I am also very concerned that my patients not have recurrences of sustained ventricular tachycardia or cardiac arrest. I believe that a successful EP result predicts that the patient will not have a recurrence at a rate that is as high as it would be if you were not able to get control in the laboratory. For me, from a pragmatic point of view, I think that is an adequate end point and for that reason I think EP testing is valuable in patients that have sustained ventricular arrhythmia. For non-sustained events, I take the opposite view point which is that I don't believe that EP testing has been tested adequately to say that it has value.

Dr. Temple: There is plenty of data showing that effective suppression followed by the use of the drug that suppressed is associated with a good prognosis. The question arises is that true true unrelated. Do you have to give the drug to get that good outcome. That question applies equally to survival or to recurrence of a bad hemodynamically unstable arrhythmia. The same question arises is it the drug or is it the ability to suppress? I don't understand why one is more confident that one has accomplished something great symptomatically if these hemodynamically unstable arrhythmias are somehow survivable I don't know why that would be, but let's say they are, I don't see where one is more comfortable in that than one is comfortable with the idea that you are actually improving survival because there is plentiful data that don't quite answer the question but give grounds for optimism. I just want to offer one thought. Many of these suppression studies have been carried out in populations that are largely or even entirely resuscitated or people who had arrhythmias that would almost surely have killed them. The mortality rate is 30-50% or something like that. When someone like Ruskin applies similar thoughts to Podrid and Lown's population, they are all very sick, when they show mortality rates in the 5% range and that applies to approximately, I don't know, say they can find suppressible regimens in half of their patients, I have the thought that that is not compatible with the results in the total population, that is they are actually treating a significant fraction of the population that has a mortality of 30-40% and they are getting only 3-4%. I don't think you can select the subgroup that will do that well. Surely we are all waiting to see what Jay Mason's study shows to pin it down in a very rigorous way, but to me, the clues are pretty good and it is not too plausible that all you are doing is identifying people who have a good prognosis.

Dr. Lipicky: I don't know that I can offer any thinking process that is useful except that I get confused a lot. I think the way to view the EPS stuff is that it is an unequivocal demonstration of antiarrhythmic activity in a patient population that basically one would want to treat with an antiarrhythmic and it is unequivocally a demonstration of antiarrhythmic activity. In people who have serious arrhythmias there are indeed many practical problems associated with doing controlled clinical trials and it is indeed fortunate that there is a wealth of data that says that if an antiarrhythmic has the ability to suppress EPS inducibility that that carries with it some predictive value that allows people to utilize a drug of that nature that has that property in a fashion that makes a difference whatever that difference may be due to. The only confusion is when one looks at EPS at a surrogate for, it is a semantic argument, it really is not a surrogate for mortality or it is not a surrogate for clinical benefit. It is an unequivocal demonstration of antiarrhythmic activity in a patient population that you otherwise would have difficulty in demonstrating the antiarrhythmic activity in. It is not controlled necessarily, but it is baseline controlled at least and in that sense it constitutes a controlled trial. It really doesn't deserve the name surrogate. I think it is the semantics of the thing.

Dr. Borer: Dr. Kowey pointed out that he finds invasive electrophysiological testing very useful clinically in patients who have a history of sustained arrhythmias. I think there is a great deal of information that indicates that if you pick out that population and you do EPS testing and you find a drug that suppresses an inducible arrhythmia that those patients do well on that drug. These patients already have been demonstrated to do poorly if nothing is done for them. I think everyone would agree to the use of EP directed drug in a patient with a history of sudden death or fainting with sustained arrhythmias. The problem is the generalizability of the finding of efficacy in that population to another population in whom you haven't done EP testing to determine whether to give them the drug or not. I think in terms of approving antiarrhythmic drugs, the utility of electrophysiologic testing would be unquestioned if you are dealing with a population that clearly has declared itself at risk. I would perhaps have some reservations, but less reservations about the approvability of a drug for suppression of arrhythmia in a population in which the drug was selected on the basis of electrophysiologic testing. I would have more reservation about identifying that population clinically without having the electrophysiologic testing done as a clinical tool in the individual patient and then giving the drug to the patient, because in an EP tested population, it worked. I think therein lies the great problem. What we are looking for is a way to generalize the applicability of the drug so that not every patient has to go through this expensive and scary invasive testing. I don't think we have reached that point yet. If you are directing the drug therapy on the basis of EP testing, you also have already shown that the proarrhythmic problem is not the problem in that patient.

Dr. Kowey: I don't know about that Jeff.

Dr. Borer: You have shown that that population with the drug selected that way does well. You can argue all you want about whether that is right. Because you gave the drug or despite the fact you gave the drug, it clearly doesn't make them worse.

Dr. Morganroth: Over the short term that you have observed them. In the past that was fine, but what about long term?

Dr. Borer: No these studies were in years.

Dr. Kowey: The reports of people who do well on EP testing run several years in many cases.

Dr. Borer: Let me back off. I said proarrhythmia, but let's say, bad outcome. You could on the basis of the electrophysiologic testing select a drug for a patient and if he felt dizzy on the drug, you could then choose to remove the drug. It seems not an unreasonable practical approach if the alternative to having a little bit of dizziness which might be due to the drug is death because of an arrhythmia that you know has a high likelihood of happening if the patient isn't on a drug. I think that we may be mixing in discussing antiarrhythmic drugs and the testing that needs to be done in order to apply them to patients. We have to be very careful to make the distinction between what we do in an individual patient and a number of tests and the type of tests we perform and the generalizability of the utility of that drug to a patient population that is defined only clinically. We have to be careful not to be overly concerned about negative effects that may not be particularly dangerous and that can be seen clinically and that can be used as the basis for withdrawing the drug if you want to.

Dr. Korakowsky: What is the possibility that the problems are related not to the drug but to the dose of the drug? Do we know that the dose response for VPC suppression and V tach suppression are the same? Is it not possible that perhaps the best study to do would be a dose response in V Tach and then decide if we really have the right dose and the right dosing interval? Perhaps that is where the problem lies?

Dr. Kowey: I think that is an excellent point. I don't think that there is any question that for particular agents, there is a definite difference in the dose that may be needed for VPD suppression versus what you need in the EP laboratory to prevent induction. The problem is that in exploring a range of doses in the EP laboratory is extremely difficult. Unless it can be done with a very short acting drug where you can change the dose or dose IV or do something innovative, you are talking about an oral dose ranging and you are looking at a broad range of doses. It is just not feasible to do that in a parallel fashion in a way that would be acceptable to an agency. You might be able to do a couple of doses, but it is very difficult to do more than that.

Dr. Korakowsky: The question is whether there are any data at all to say that it is the same or that it is not the same? If is a query as to methodology. If you can feel comfortable with the methodology, you would want a small number of patients. If the methodology seems to be totally wrong, doing a lot of patients, getting a lot of garbage data, is not going to help you.

Dr. Lipicky: I don't think there is any data that directly

compares it.

Dr. Kowey: I think that for a drug like propafenone that the doses that are required for non-inducibility in the electrophysiology laboratory tend to be at the much higher end of their dose range versus their VPB effect.

Dr. Lipicky: Is this at steady state or is this acute test?

Dr. Kowey: This is after people have been on the dose for several days.

Dr. Morganroth: That may be because the drug is not terribly effective in that population or because if you take other drugs like encainide and flecainide, what was learned there was that one had to use much smaller doses and let them go to steady state before changing that dose or your rate of proarrhythmic death could be very high.

Dr. Temple: That is very different. What you found there was that people with bad hearts couldn't tolerate doses that people with VPB's and presumably better hearts could, but they also weren't terribly successful in the EP laboratory either.

Dr. Morganroth: They were as successful as propafenone if not more so in terms of the percent of the patients rendered non-inducible.

Dr. Temple: Yes, but most of them aren't as successful as procainamide for example.

Dr. Morganroth: They are pretty comparable. The encainide and flecainide data bases have about a 20-30% success rate of non-inducibility.

Dr. Lipicky: It depends on who you talk to. Some of the EP people say that they would never choose encainide and flecainide on the basis of EP testing because it basically is not predictive and the return rate is so low that it is not useful to take those into the laboratory.

Dr. Temple: I think it is the second point that is the one that is most important.

Dr. Lipicky: That is correct. An error in my language.

Dr. Morganroth: The question asked is do we know about the dose of the antiarrhythmic drug as defined in the PVC populations and how that relates to the EP population and my answer would be that you don't. I gave an example of drugs that show this point perhaps on the basis of their tolerability.

Dr. Temple: There isn't one dose. My impression is that for every drug we know about, they overlap. The kinds of doses that you use for VPB's are the same kinds of doses you leave people on. That is not terrific guidance if the dose range is 4 or 5 fold, but they are sort of in the same neighborhood. One isn't an order of magnitude different from the other.

Dr. Kowey: You are right I think, but when we look at new drugs we are finding a fairly low non-inducibility rate with these compounds and sometimes I really wonder if the reason why we are seeing that isn't because we have gotten a dose range from a different subset of patients and we apply that dose range in the EP population. Of course there are issues of tolerance, and that is a totally different issue, but I sometimes wonder if we are not orders of magnitude off from the correct dose for non-inducibility because we have been misled by our VPB trials.

Dr. Temple: You have to find a drug where you can push the dose without doing devastating harm. We thought of EP testing to be a forecast at least as evidence that this drug can be useful. It is quite true, we didn't go on to say it is useful only when you use it in the EP lab and direct therapy that way. It was taken as evidence that this was a drug that at least in some people would be of value. Dr. Borer raises the question of whether all you really know is if you use it just that way, it's valuable. Certainly labeling is not written that way. We considered that was just too wonderful a thing to do for the EP people and never were quite as directive as that. We didn't try to settle the issue of Holter versus PES but you raise the question and I think it is worth discussing whether all we really know is that this is one safe and probably effective way to use it and you really don't know whether Holter directed therapy with the same drug is safe or effective.

Dr. Packer: I think that EP is certainly a much better guide than Holter, but I am still not convinced that it is not a surrogate end point. It is a surrogate end point. It is a way of judging activity of a drug. It is not really a way of judging efficacy. Efficacy says you have fewer sudden deaths and you have fewer episodes of syncope. That is efficacy. Activity is suppression of an inducible arrhythmia, so I think it still falls into the realm of a surrogate end point. Having said that, it doesn't mean that it is not an acceptable surrogate end point, but it is still a surrogate end point.

Dr. Temple: Many people think it is a an accurate, valid surrogate end point. The fly in the ointment is whether what you are learning is not that use of the drug directed in this manner can prove survival, but rather that people who are capable of responding to this drug by suppressing have a good survival whether you give them a drug or not.

Dr. Packer: If you define surrogate as a laboratory or clinical testing phenomenon, that is used to judge whether a drug would work to reduce clinically relevant end points then it is a surrogate end point, and it could be a very acceptable surrogate end point but it is still a surrogate end point.

Dr. Temple: Just as decreased blood pressure is a surrogate end point for decreased risk of stroke. Everyone seems to believe that.

Dr. Morganroth: Well there are good trials to suggest that. Dr. Lipicky didn't agree. He thought it wasn't a surrogate end point.

Dr. Lipicky: It is not clear to me that the discussion is useful at all as to whether it is surrogate end point or not. Everybody talking about it agrees that it demonstrates antiarrhythmic activity and everybody talking agrees that it probably is useful in some predictive way in some general sense. It is not necessary to agree that it is or is not a surrogate. The issue I guess is that really needs some agreement or discussion is whether because it is a critical piece of evidence in people with serious arrhythmias and whether in fact one has to incorporate that empirical information about that piece of evidence, into labeling because in fact one doesn't have the ability to extrapolate beyond it and that is probably more germane to discussions about antiarrhythmic agents and their approvability than agreement as to whether it is a surrogate for mortality end point because it clearly demonstrates that it is an antiarrhythmic drug.

Dr. Temple: But so does VPB suppression and we have been shaken in our belief that that is a useful indicator.

Dr. Lipicky: No. Not at all. I still accept that as a totally useful criteria to make the decision that this is an antiarrhythmic agent. It however is clear from other information that VPB suppression per se should not be encouraged as a use of antiarrhythmics and therefore that doesn't help me make a decision that this antiarrhythmic is approvable because it clearly demonstrates it is an antiarrhythmic, so what?

Dr. Morganroth: The so what relates to benefit, right? There are two issues, activity and benefit to the patient. There is no question that everyone on this panel I suspect would agree that whether one uses Holter for PVC patients of EP for sustained VT patients that if the drug gets rid of the PVC's on the Holter or the inducibility of sustained VT that the drug has activity and it is thus an antiarrhythmic drug. The next question is, so what?

Dr. Lipicky: But that in fact is where the difference comes.

Dr. Morganroth: On Holter, we used to think that Holter was a surrogate end point for something and now CAST says maybe it is a surrogate end point for death more than anything else. So no longer will Dr. Lipicky accept Holter activity as "benefit" for the patient. Clearly if you reduce the ability to induce sustained VT by EPS that shows the drug has activity in that model. The real question is, is that end point, lack of inducibility by EP, a surrogate end point for benefit to the patient?

Dr. Lipicky: I stop my thinking process right there. That is, it is clear demonstration in a patient population in which it could potentially be used that it works.

Dr. Latts: To clarify the question, Dr. Lipicky, suppose we brought you an NDA of a drug that had been worked up by PES only. We never did PVC studies. We showed in 15% it suppresses inducibility. We did long term follow-up on those patients and we have a reasonable safety data base, is that an approval drug?

Dr. Lipicky: That requires a couple of days. No, I don't think so. I don't think so because there are many aspects of the drug that have been defined and that information alone would be insufficient to be able to come to grips with the properties of the drug.

Dr. Packer: But Dr. Lipicky, if you said that is an efficacy end point and if a sponsor decided that the only appropriate use of an antiarrhythmic drug is in an EP laboratory but that no physician should give the antiarrhythmic drug outside an EP laboratory and if you were to implode the entire field of antiarrhythmic or drug therapy into a kernel of people who were going to definitely benefit from the drug and they studied it only in that patient population using the appropriate methods, then that is all you would need.

Dr. Lipicky: I would still have major troubles because I don't necessarily believe that the drug would be used only within those limited constraints. There would be a lack of information with respect to why the drug should be used only within those constraints and not outside of those constraints and so from my vantage point, that would be devoid of a bunch of information. Now one might be able to push the legal issue, and say, well but you have no legal basis for not approving that and that would be a pretty powerful argument, but it doesn't detract from the fact that that would be a totally inadequate data base and it would be a totally inadequate description of the chemical compound and that it would be very discomforting to think that one might have to act positively.

Dr. Temple: Maybe the question that is being asked is suppose the only effectiveness data came from that setting and apart from that the usual pharmacokinetics, maybe a little dose response in VPB rates just so you know where to start, but not the usual 300 patient comparison with quinidine.

Dr. Lipicky: That is fine. That is a non-useful comparison anyhow.

Dr. Temple: Yes, but it gets you certain safety information I think you can argue for. I think the premise was agreed to that that could be the major effectiveness data.

Dr. Lipicky: That could be the major effectiveness data but it can't be the only data in the application.

Dr. Packer: But are we convinced that having said that and let's say you build an NDA entirely around an EP guided data base, and have all the pharmacokinetics and the safety data and you had exposed it to an adequate number of patients, and it wasn't the only thing in the NDA but it was certainly the pivotal part of the efficacy section of the NDA, and in fact the sponsor agreed that together with all the other people interested in antiarrhythmic drug therapy to mount a major educational campaign in the United States that asymptomatic PVC's should not be treated and that the only people who should receive antiarrhythmic drugs should be done in the EP lab under the guidelines, that would be an approvable NDA.

Dr. Lipicky: Yes, sure. If you look back through the questions that have been asked of the advisory committee at the approval of every antiarrhythmic that has ever been done so far in the last six years, there has never been a question that asked whether it was effective.

Dr. Morganroth: I have a problem with this. You are willing to approve this antiarrhythmic application that just outlined on the basis of demonstrating only activity without any data demonstrating benefit to the patient. That is, Dr. Packer didn't propose that you show decreased syncope or decreased mortality. The reason you accepted that I think is that you perceived that population studied by EP data to have a very high potential for benefit by having their arrhythmia suppressed. Since the potential benefit is high, you are willing to accept any potential risk that is not well defined thus accepting EP as a surrogate end point for benefit.

Dr. Lipicky: No, you have taken away some information from Dr. Packer's NDA that could have been in there..

Dr. Morganroth: That he didn't express.

Dr. Lipicky: He didn't say it would not have data regarding whether people fainted or not.

Dr. Morganroth: So you would demand that his NDA, that there be benefit data.

Dr. Temple: I think you would follow up those patients. Confirm the expected observation that they did well.

Dr. Morganroth: Did well compared to what?

Dr. Temple: Compared to what you expect them to do. You are not going to have a control group.

Dr. Lipicky: Baseline control is fine in a population of that ilk.

Dr. Temple: You would expect a low mortality which is what the system predicts, low occurrence rate.

Dr. Temple: You have to study a range of the population you are talking about just as you do now.
Dr. Morganroth: So historical controls would still be OK in a population that has high risk. So if I took a population of patients with non-sustained VT with EF's under 30% in which their risk of sudden death may be extremely high, maybe in the order of 20%, or if I took congestive cardiomyopathy patients with non-sustained VT at a similar risk and I showed by following those patients with no placebo controlled group that their benefit was that they only had a 3% or 4% mortality in that next year, would that be sufficient to demonstrate benefit?
Dr. Lipicky: That population would be suitable to study. EPS data in that population would be useful from the vantage point of gaining approvability and the experiential part of what you would observe in studying that population would be useful from the vantage point of gaining approvability but I don't think it is in the context that you are portraying it of being that information alone is sufficient.
Dr. Morganroth: It would make it sufficient if it was studied by EP instead of Holter.
Dr. Lipicky: I think you need EP in there somewhere.
Dr. Kowey: I think we better go back a little bit because we have totally shifted the population. I think the NDA that Dr. Packer was describing did not have that population in it, did it Milton?
Dr. Packer: That is right. The NDA I was describing was only a patient population that had died previously but had had a sustained hemodynamically significant arrhythmia and in fact one could say that of all the patient populations for whom antiarrhythmic therapy may be targeted. That is one population everyone agrees should be targeted for antiarrhythmic drug therapy, so if you confined the whole NDA to a patient population as you said, I think it is perfectly reasonable for a sponsor to say, "Look, we don't know what antiarrhythmic drugs do to people with benign PVC's or simple complex PVC's." We don't know what antiarrhythmic drug therapy does to non-sustained ventricular tachycardia that is asymptomatic. We do know that there is a mandate from the cardiology community to treat people who have had hemodynamically significant sustained VT and VF. We want to develop a drug only for those people for whom, despite the fact that it is a very small market comparatively, we think that is the only population for whom benefit is perceived to be present and we only want to develop a drug for that patient population. That wouldn't be such a bad idea.
Dr. Borer: I think that the non-sustained VT population with low ejection fraction for sure is a patient population that is at high risk. Other than the use of vasodilating drugs, in that population as a whole, I am not aware of any data that suggests that any therapy, any management strategy that we have ever attempted has any benefit in prolonging life in that patient population and I certainly think that it would be very difficult for the FDA to approve an antiarrhythmic drug in a population defined on the basis of structural heart disease, poor systolic function and non-sustained VT because of directed data alone. There just isn't the data base to justify that kind of action without a follow-up showing that there is indeed statistically significant clinical benefit when you follow that management strategy.

Dr. Morganroth: That is a controlled mortality trial.
Dr. Borer: That is right.
Dr. Morganroth: You would have to have a reference group and that essentially is what now is being done in CAST or in other potential mortality trials using a higher risk group. Is there a claim potential for symptomatic ventricular arrhythmia alone?
Dr. Lipicky: You would have to evaluate the risk benefit.
Dr. Temple: In people with what underlying arrhythmia.
Dr. Morganroth: The indication could read "The antiarrhythmic drug is useful in preventing or eliminating debilitating symptomatic ventricular arrhythmias" and those ventricular arrhythmias are PVC's or and non-sustained VT in patients with normal hearts or with structural heart disease. The benefit to the population being elimination of symptoms and the risk has to be clarified. That is, one would have to show that the drug didn't cause increased mortality for example. Does it have to show it doesn't increase mortality? Could it show that it was just neutral? That is, take a data base like sotalol or moricizine and let's assume they had a very clear study that demonstrated that they could eliminate symptoms in a few patients.
Dr. Temple: And they had a CAST study or something that didn't make things worse.
Dr. Morganroth: And they had a CAST study or post-infarction mortality trial like the sotalol NDA may have. Let's assume for the sake of this discussion they have data that show that the drug doesn't increase mortality, and they show the benefit and they work out all the pharmacology, have an EP data base, etc. Should they get a claim for symptomatic arrhythmias?
Dr. Temple: Sure. It is going to be increasingly hard to get that kind of background data. People aren't doing placebo controlled post-infarction trials anymore very often with beta blockers, so sotalol could be the last one through on that and moricizine had the good fortune to be the other drug in CAST.
Dr. Morganroth: But let's say that happens and you end up approving both or either of those agents with the "old" claims: symptomatic ventricular arrhythmias and life-threatening ventricular arrhythmias. Now a new drug comes on the scene that is in development and it wants the same claim because that is a pretty big market. They want to compete in that market, and they want of course then to show that they don't increase mortality. How do they do that because it would be unethical to study that same population with a placebo control?
Dr. Lipicky: Do a positive controlled trial.
Dr. Kowey: If you show any antiarrhythmic drug reduces mortality and you define a patient population who should receive that drug which was studied in the trial that showed a reduction in mortality, then it would be unethical to withdraw that drug. Everyone in that patient population should receive the drug, then the ethical thing is to study another. If you think there is a possible incremental benefit, then you study it on top of everyone receiving that baseline drug, dropping the placebo controlled fashion. Alternatively, you do an active controlled study of sufficient numbers. It is very difficult.
Dr. Temple: The method of control is a difficult question. It depends a little on what you are trying to show. If someone offered

us an active controlled post-infarction beta blocker study, we would reject it. Of all the trials of that kind that have been done against placebo, only 3 or 4 have actually shown a significant difference from placebo and very good sized well conducted trials have failed to distinguish drug from placebo. So you can't learn about effectiveness, but you are raising a different question. Can you learn about non-harm by doing a large enough study and ruling out major damage? I wonder, maybe you could.

Dr. Lipicky: Generally speaking, when I have heard that issue discussed, people are generally satisfied with something like no more than 50% more or something on that order, and therefore someone isn't looking for 10 and 15% differences in rates and positive controlled trials are capable of having sufficient power to be able to give one assurances with respect to those kinds of limits. Indeed, if one were thinking in terms of 10% or 15%, then probably you would start getting into the proportions where it was not practical to really think one could derive that information.

Dr. Moore: One possibility for these patients who are very high risk for a placebo group would be of course to use an AICD and how large a trial would you then need to prove efficacy?

Dr. Kowey: The answer to your extremely important question, is the real current technology, although it is soon to be outdated, doesn't allow those kinds of trials very easily because of the fact that many of the people receive an appropriate device discharges, and it is very hard to do a valid study to count events in these patients. In fact the latest look at the AICD literature mainly from CPI indicates that at least 30 to 40 and maybe even 50% of the shocks that are delivered to the patients are inappropriate, by whatever we can use as an appropriate determination. That is, the patient did not have the typical symptom, etc. With the newer devices in which there will be abilities to interrogate and in which there will be memory loops so that we can actually pull information off the device, it will be possible perhaps to do these kinds of trials. The answer to your question about how many patients really depends on the kinds of patients that you select, and there are may patients with devices who have fairly frequent recurrences.

Dr. Temple: No. The reports by people like Ruskin have taken people who don't have obvious anything on their Holter but who have had an episode of sudden death and have been resuscitated, they then follow them for a period of a year or so and what they find is that the re-occurrence rate, either death or something, they get resuscitated for, is 20 or 30 or 40% and in the people they can't find a suppressing drug for and it is very low in the people that they do.

Dr. Kowey: But that is not the population you are putting devices in. That is a different population. The way the device is handled these days, is if you think a patient is going to have frequent recurrences, you don't put the device in.

Dr. Temple: That is what I am describing. A person who has nothing much on Holter but is inducible and has had a death.

Dr. Kowey: Right, they will have an event, but only 50% of the people will shock in the first year.

Dr. Temple: That is O.K. Fifty versus zero is easy to interpret.

Dr. Kowey: If you have a drug that completely suppresses the events. It depends on the power of the event.

Dr. Temple: It isn't the drug. It is you will only use the drug if you succeeded in suppressing EP inducibility.

Dr. Kowey: That is adding in another factor which is the fact that you have tested the drug in the laboratory in addition to putting the device in. That is a different study. We are talking about a population of patients who get a defibrillator and then without any regard of whether you get an effect or not, I mean either design is appropriate.

Dr. Temple: The great thing about this is you can find out that the drug might work and then not give it.

Dr. Kowey: Absolutely true. That would be a more elegant design, but in a simpler study, it would simply be giving the patient the drug or not giving him the drug.

Dr. Temple: With unselected therapy, who knows what you might find. You might find that you make them worse. It seems to me that the study could be very small.

Dr. Kowey: If you pick the patients appropriately, yes. I guess that is what I was saying, that it really is patient population dependent and how you select that patient population.

Dr. Philip DeVane: Experience from clinical practice I think suggests that electrophysiologists recognize not just complete suppression of inducibility but also an intermediate form. I think work by Len Horowitz has suggested that patients do better although they continue to have events and the implication being that they would continue on the test medication but still have events. The discussion has talked about suppression of inducibility or not, but is there an intermediate form, and would this be a basis for approval of a drug?

Dr. Temple: Dr. Horowitz's observations are mostly with amiodarone where he thought there was an intermediate stage where you recurred but didn't die. I am not sure that people believe that is true for other situations and I am not sure that everybody believes that for amiodarone.

Dr. Borer: But nonetheless, that is a question to be tested, which presumably ought to be done if someone though that there as benefit to a drug that could do this kind of thing. You would take a patient population, give it and see if there was indeed a reduction of badness in that group, however you choose to define it.

Dr. Kowey: I think that would be probably *de facto* a part of any of these trials, for if you are just looking at non-inducibility obviously you will never gather enough patients for adequate follow-up, so that *de facto* you would end up with a population of patients who had an intermediate outcome and I will tell you, just from the scientific point of view, I would be extremely interested in knowing that data for any agent, other than amiodarone. I think that is the best tested drug, because for example there are some data with propafenone again, that indicates that a clear Holter and slowing of VT in the lab doesn't only cause non-lethal events, it reduces overall events. Whether that is drug specific or specific to a class or whatever, we don't know. I think it is an extremely interesting and a very important part of any of those trials such as Dr. Packer described.

Dr. Packer: Given that as a background, just one question, which is very much related. If all the decision making is potentially based on EP testing, for people who have an established requirement for an effective antiarrhythmic drug, is it uncertain why that should not be something that is not incorporated in labeling?

Dr. Temple: I think it is a very good question. In the past, it was considered one additional kind of evidence of antiarrhythmogenicity and in particular in a population that was very much of interest, people with bad disease, but it didn't lead to the conclusion that was the only way to use it. If that is the only thing we really feel comfortable with, I mean there is obviously another side that will come out and say, "Oh we don't have to do that, we could learn the same thing from the right kind of exercise testing for example where the Lown-Podrid data is at least 2/3 exercise testing with similar good results". So I think there are people who would argue that EP testing is not the only way to fix on a good prognosis but is one way. That would be our reluctance, we would be sort of settling a scientific controversy in labeling. It is not necessarily our role.

Dr. Morganroth: But if the Calgary data and ESVEM come out the same way, what do you think?

Dr. Temple: I think then you have a very strong case.

Dr. Borer: But even without those data, the fact is if the data you have that allow somebody to safely and effectively use a drug indicate that you can do that, if you have EP testing and there are not other data that are presented that show you how you could use the drug, then the FDA wouldn't be settling any kind of scientific controversy. It would just be supporting the validity of data that have been presented to it. One could then go on and devise a different strategy of testing, demonstrate that it works and have the FDA change the label.

Dr. Lipicky: Let me put in a dissenting voice. Let's say for example one had an antihypertensive drug that got worked up in people who were appropriately renin classified and what one found was that it lowered blood pressure more in the high renin group than in the low renin group, in fact the low renin group did not meet placebo. Would that lead to explicit instructions for use that said, "You must bring people into the hospital. You must deplete them of salt. You must do renin testing and then you must only employ this drug in patients that have been thusly screened" etc.

Dr. Temple: Yes, that is the example you gave.

Dr. Lipicky: I don't think it would, because it doesn't have the same mystique.

Dr. Temple: There is another reason. The cost of trying an anti-hypertensive drug and finding that it doesn't work is not very great and you might conclude that it still might be reasonable to try it out. You might. But in the arrhythmia case, that is not such a good idea. The therapeutic trial you give results in death if you make a mistake.

Dr. Lipicky: But how do you know that. It could still be that people picked by other methods do better than placebo.

Dr. Temple: In the case you describe, what happens when you give it someone with low renin is that he doesn't get a response. you learn that in a week or two and you then give him another drug. No big deal.

Dr. Lipicky: Oh no, they get some. Enough to satisfy the clinician.

Dr. Temple: In that case there is no particular problem at all, and you don't necessarily say that you must do renin status on these people.

Dr. Lipicky: Yes right, but all things can potentially have relative efficacy.

Dr. Temple: All right, but if you go to the arrhythmia case, you were worried that these drugs actually make people worse at least in some cases.

Dr. Lipicky: I am not, you are.

Dr. Temple: You're not?

Dr. Lipicky: That is not my worry, so don't put that into your thinking process.

Dr. Temple: If I thought that antiarrhythmics were at worse neutral, I think we would have a very different sort of way to think and I don't think that is tenable anymore. They are not at worse neutral. They are at worse, deadly, so that choosing one in a way that seems likely to make it a value seems particularly important here.

Dr. Lipicky: Oh I see.

Dr. Temple: The idea that the major effect on this data would be EPS directed shouldn't exclude the thought that you would actually do a little more than we now see. For example, I would think that the patients in whom therapy was chosen that way would be followed for a period of time to kind of confirm that nothing terrible happens.

Dr. Morganroth: By an active control instead of just an open label?

Dr. Temple: Ideally, that is what you would like, even if you didn't try to randomize the order, but there is no reason not to do that actually, you would take a group of people and do the usual drug search for them and you would put the ones on your drug on and you would also follow up the experience in the patients who turned out to suppress with some other drug than yours and follow the people who didn't suppress at all.

Dr. Morganroth: So it is open label, follow all groups. Now that is very different from the kind of studies that are now being conducted, or you have asked them to conduct which are double blind, positive controlled, studies with long term follow up.

Dr. Temple: That would be better. If you could find people who suppress on more than one drug, you could introduce randomization.

Dr. Morganroth: What the agency has most recently recommended from what I understand is the requirement of positive controlled, EP trials in which patients with inducible sustained VT are randomized once they are inducible to drug X or drug Y.

Dr. Temple: Wait a minute, without showing suppression?

Dr. Morganroth: No, they could randomize to drug X or drug Y, then they are given drug X or drug Y, another EP test is done to define if the patients are non-inducible.

Dr. Lipicky: Let me tell you what the rest of the study covered. If one of the drugs was considered to be very unsafe and the question was to evaluate the relative safety of the two drugs in two settings. One setting was in the acute loading circumstance where in fact people get into trouble when they are doing EPS and the second circumstance was during basically a positive control parallel trial that had EP used as its means of getting people on to drug because this was in patients with serious arrhythmias.

Dr. Morganroth: And what value do you see from that data in terms of understanding the new drug?

Dr. Lipicky: Relative safety.

Dr. Morganroth: Relative safety compared to a drug that you know is bad in that setting so it is to sort of make you comfortable that it is still good or to see that it is in fact equally bad.

Dr. Lipicky: Or that it is worse.

Dr. Morganroth: So it is a safety comparison more than an efficacy.

Dr. Temple: Ray, would you describe that trial exactly.

Dr. Lipicky: People with bad arrhythmias come in and are randomized with respect to the time that two drugs would be administered for purposes of EPS.

Dr. Temple: And they are never going to get anymore than 2 drugs? Two drugs is all they get a crack at? Do they get another drug if they fail on the first?

Dr. Lipicky: No and the first drug that they are suppressible by...

Dr. Temple: They are only getting one drug.

Dr. Lipicky: No, which drug they are going to get. They are patients who must be treated so that they are going to receive one of these two drugs if they are EPS suppressible by one or the other.

Dr. Temple: So they are getting both?

Dr. Lipicky: No they will receive one of the two if they are EPS suppressible by either one, so that the first randomization is that is the order in which one would receive the drug.

Dr. Temple: So they are getting both?

Dr. Lipicky: No, any one patient will only receive one drug if the first drug administered suppresses.

Dr. Temple: All right, that is fine. They get the other one if it doesn't though?

Dr. Lipicky: Yes.

Dr. Morganroth: No, there is no crossover.

Dr. Lipicky: No, these are people who have to leave the hospital on treatment so if the first drug doesn't suppress them, they have to get another drug.

Dr. Kowey: Not the other drug in the study.

Dr. Lipicky: Why not?

Dr. Kowey: No I am asking you the design. It is the other drug in the study?

Dr. Lipicky: Yes.

Dr. Kowey: So they do get crossed over?

Dr. Lipicky: Yes, but everyone does not get crossed over.

Dr. Morganroth: Only the half that are on the experimental arm would have the choice of getting the approved drug, because the patients who were initially randomized to the approved drug would not have the availability of the non-approved drug.

Dr. Temple: The point of that randomization is that there is a presumption that failing on one therapy might mean that you are different from someone who hasn't failed on therapy. So randomizing the order is to give each of the drugs a crack at the more virginal patient.

Dr. Moore: As you can see, every time we talk about antiarrhythmics, we present more questions than answers.

13

HOW TO DEMONSTRATE THE EFFICACY OF A NEW DRUG FOR THE TREATMENT OF CHRONIC HEART FAILURE

MILTON PACKER, M.D.

Center for Heart Failure Research, Division of Cardiology
Mount Sinai School of Medicine, New York, NY

Several approaches are possible in the design of a research plan for the purpose of gaining approval for a new agent for the treatment of chronic heart failure. Any successful research plan, however, must show (with a reasonable degree of confidence) that the new agent is effective and safe for the treatment of this condition.

All claims of efficacy must be based on data derived from double-blind, placebo-controlled trials. Although such a requirement is absolute, the design of such trials remains flexible. The trial may be a treatment trial (i.e., the new drug is added to medical regimen) or a withdrawal trial (i.e., all patients are treated with the new drug, which is then blindly withdrawn in some). The trial may require no background therapy or may permit (or mandate) background treatment with digitalis, diuretics and/or a converting-enzyme inhibitor.

The syndrome of heart failure can be defined as exercise intolerance due to dyspnea and/or fatigue that can be physiologically related to an identifiable abnormality of cardiac function. The abnormality of cardiac function may be ventricular or valvular; if ventricular, it may primarily affect systolic or diastolic performance. Hence, the heart failure state has two components: (1) a symptom complex and (2) an abnormality of cardiac function. In general, there is a poor relation between the severity of the symptom complex and the severity of cardiac dysfunction. Of the two, the clinical definition of heart failure relies more heavily on the symptom complex, and hence, measures of the symptom complex (morbidity and mortality) provide the primary measures of efficacy. In contrast, measures of cardiac function are secondary measures of efficacy.

PRIMARY ENDPOINTS

To gain approval for a new agent for heart failure, the drug must be shown to make patients feel better or live longer (or both). No other measures of efficacy are presently recognized as surrogate endpoints.

Four clinically relevant endpoints may be evaluated in trials of patients with heart failure: (1) a reduction in symptoms; (2) an improvement in exercise tolerance; (3) a reduction in morbidity (rate of worsening heart failure); (4) a reduction in mortality. The first three endpoints are commonly grouped together and assessed in the same studies, since they reflect different approaches to evaluating how patients with heart failure feel. In contrast, the fourth endpoint (i.e., mortality) is commonly evaluated independently of the other three, since much larger numbers of patients need to be studied and the effect of a drug on mortality may bear little relation to its effect on symptoms, exercise tolerance and morbidity. In general, it is helpful for a new agent to demonstrate an beneficial effect with respect to as many of these endpoints as possible. In addition, reasonable evidence should be provided that the drug does not affect any of these endpoints in an adverse fashion.

Reduction in symptoms

The most straight-forward means of determining that a drug exerts a favorable effect on the syndrome of heart failure is by means of questions directed at assessing the severity of specific symptoms. Both symptoms and the patient's sense of well-being can be measured by either a categorical approach or visual analog scale and should reflect the viewpoints of both the patient and the investigator. Although a variety of "quality of life" instruments have been proposed (nearly every trial has used a different questionnaire), none has yet been validated and none has been shown to reflect the severity of the heart failure syndrome better than direct questions concerning specific symptoms.

Improvement in exercise tolerance

An essential part of any heart failure trial design is an assessment of exercise capacity. This assessment provides an objective and quantifiable measure of a critical feature of the heart failure syndrome (i.e., exercise intolerance). The exercise test may be maximal or submaximal, may evaluate peak effort or endurance. and may or may not be guided by direct measurements of respiratory gas exchange. There is no evidence that one approach to exercise is superior to any other.

All exercise testing in heart failure is associated with a predictable placebo response, i.e., an increase in exercise duration with placebo in the absence of any change in active therapy. The magnitude of this response may be so large so as to obscure any increment in exercise tolerance that may be due to the new drug. This may explain why many effective drugs for heart failure do not reproducibly distinguish themselves from placebo in trials that use exercise tolerance as the only endpoint.

Any effort to minimize the placebo effect will reduce the variance of the measurement and enhance the ability to demonstrate a difference between active drug and placebo. Recent evidence indicates that the placebo effect can be decreased by repeated exercise during the single-blind run-in period of the trial. Five years ago (when a single baseline exercise test was commonly employed in trials, the placebo effect over 12 weeks averaged about 150 seconds. More recently, when the criteria were narrowed to require two tests within 15%, the placebo effect was reduced to about 60-70 seconds over 12 weeks. More recently, we have developed a new criterion for baseline reproducibility (3 tests within 60 seconds without a trend) which has reduced the placebo effect to 30-35 seconds in a multicenter trial and only 6 seconds in a single-center study (1). This new criterion should enhance the ability to distinguish an active drug from placebo using relatively small numbers of patients.

Reduction in Morbidity

The ability of a drug to reduce the incidence of worsening heart failure during long-term follow-up provides a compelling case for the efficacy of a new drug for heart failure. In this regard, the criteria to be used to define "worsening" need to be prospectively stated. They may include (but not be limited to): (1) the need for hospitalization or emergency room visit for worsening symptoms; or (2) the need for additional therapy (i.e., vasodilators, increasing diuretics, intravenous inotropic drugs, etc). Unfortunately, the criteria for transplantation are too variable to permit this event to be used as a criterion for increased morbidity.

Combined Endpoints and Endpoint Interactions

Because symptom scores, exercise testing and morbidity evaluations provide different measures of the same process, all three are commonly included in pivotal trials to provide a complete measure of drug efficacy. In general, a trial provides strong support for an approvable NDA if all three endpoints show favorable directional changes, which reach (or almost reach) statistical significance at the $P < 0.05$ level. For example, if in a trial of 250 subjects, patients treated with a new drug show an improvement in symptom scores ($P < 0.05$) and in morbidity ($P < 0.05$), an increase in exercise tolerance at a significance level between 0.10 and 0.05 still provides strong evidence for efficacy. Similarly, the finding of an improvement in exercise tolerance ($P < 0.05$) with trends towards improved symptom score ($P < 0.10$) and morbidity ($P < 0.15$) may also stand as a pivotal trial of efficacy.

Considerable doubts, however, can be raised if the directional changes with respect to all three key variables are not concordant. For example, one should be concerned about studies, in which exercise tolerance improves on active drug ($P < 0.05$), but the number of patients who drop out because of worsening heart failure is greater on active drug than on placebo. Such a result suggests that the improvement in exercise capacity in patients assigned to active therapy was the result of the drop out of large numbers of nonresponders. Similarly, one should be wary of studies, in which exercise tolerance improves, but symptom scores deteriorate.

All three primary endpoints need not be evaluated in every pivotal study. An improvement in exercise tolerance in a small study (n=20 or 30) can provide important evidence for efficacy, but such small numbers of patients cannot provide information concerning morbidity. Conversely, a large study (n=1000) designed to evaluate morbidity over long periods of time need not incorporate measures of exercise tolerance, if the reduction in morbidity is unequivocal. Hence, either exercise tolerance or morbidity can be the primary endpoint in a pivotal study. However, symptom scores alone should not be relied upon as the only evidence for efficacy; instead, symptoms scores can support a primary demonstration of benefit based on either enhanced exercise tolerance or reduced morbidity.

Reduction in Mortality

If a mortality claim is being sought, the effect of the new drug on mortality should be evaluated in a large, prospectively designed study. If a mortality claim is not being sought, the safety of the drug (with respect to survival) should be estimated by combining the mortality data from all of the short-term, placebo-controlled efficacy studies.

The sponsor should not attempt to gauge the effect of a drug on survival by comparing the observed mortality in open-label studies with that predicted (using data from the literature) for a patient cohort with baseline characteristics similar to that exposed to the new drug. Such estimates generally overestimate the mortality in the cohort being identified and cannot be used to provide reasonable reassurances about the absence or presence of a mortality effect.

SECONDARY ENDPOINTS

Invasive and noninvasive measures of cardiac function are secondary endpoints of interest in the approval of a new drug for heart failure. Of the two, invasive measurements provide more important support for efficacy than noninvasive estimates of systolic function.

Invasive hemodynamic testing

Because most patients with heart failure have low values for cardiac output and elevated values for ventricular filling pressures at rest or during exercise, it would seem logical to evaluate the efficacy of therapeutic interventions based on their ability to correct the hemodynamic abnormalities seen in patients with this disorder.

Pitfalls of hemodynamic measurements. Unfortunately, in the absence of a control group, investigators cannot be certain that the hemodynamic changes seen after the administration of a new agent represent a true drug effect (2). Spontaneous fluctuations are frequently seen in the absence of drug therapy and can be interpreted as reaching statistical (and biological) significance, if postdrug effects are not assessed at fixed times and if threshold values (that exceed the level of spontaneous variability) are not used to rule out time-related rather than drug-related effects. If an investigator defines a "peak effect" independently for each variable regardless of the time of occurrence, he creates a self-fulfilling prophecy that a true drug effect has occurred. Even if uniform times and threshold values are used, hemodynamic changes mimicking a beneficial drug response may be seen in the absence of effective drug therapy, if measurements are performed immediately after right heart catheterization or after the ingestion of a meal (3). In particular, intravascular instrumentation appears to elicit notable systemic vasoconstriction (presumably related to overt or unapparent anxiety), which dissipates in 12 to 24 hours. If predrug measurements are performed during this immediate postcatheterization period, any subsequent measurements performed weeks or months later can be interpreted as showing beneficial effects, if such long-term measurements are compared with the initial artifactually vasoconstricted state; similar degrees of systemic vasoconstriction may not be provoked during a second invasive study. If precautions are not taken, investigators may report the occurrence of sustained hemodynamic benefits in patients receiving ineffective treatment.

Initial vs long-term hemodynamic effects. To make matters more complicated, there appears to be a very complex relation between the short- and long-term effects of drug used in the treatment of heart failure. The immediate benefits seen with some agents may not be sustained during long-term treatment, because the pharmacologic actions of the drug become attenuated with time. Conversely, some patients who fail to show any hemodynamic response to the initial administration of a new therapeutic agent may show gradual improvement with time, because prolonged exposure to the drug sets into motion changes that progressively enhance the responsiveness of the circulation to treatment. Consequently, because the long-term effects of therapy bear a variable and unpredictable relation to to the initial response to treatment, the potential long-term efficacy of any therapeutic intervention cannot be assessed by testing the hemodynamic response to only the first dose of a new drug (4,5).

Role of hemodynamic measurements. Despite the pitfalls noted above, the demonstration that a new drug produces long-term hemodynamic benefits provides substantial (although not pivotal) support for the efficacy of the agent for the treatment of heart failure. In addition, such studies demonstrate which doses of the new drug are likely to be effective in pivotal trials (see above) and form the physiologic basis for how the new drug can favorably affect symptoms and exercise tolerance.

Noninvasive Measures of Left Ventricular Function

Although a variety of noninvasive techniques can provide objective, quantifiable and reproducible measures of cardiac performance, many drugs for the treatment of heart failure produce marked hemodynamic and clinical improvement without a notable changes in noninvasive indexes. Most of the changes seen in these noninvasive measures are quite small and fall within the range of error for many of these measurements. Furthermore, conventional imaging techniques only reflect changes in systolic function; they do not quantify alterations in mitral or aortic regurgitant flow or in ventricular diastolic function, both of which may contribute significantly to the hemodynamic improvement seen during effective treatment. Conversely, changes in noninvasive measures of left ventricular performance seen during the course of effective drug therapy have not been shown to correlate closely with observed changes in hemodynamic variables (measured invasively), clinical status or functional capacity (6). In fact, the left ventricular ejection fraction may increase significantly in patients with heart failure whose clinical state has deteriorated during treatment and who have fared worse than their placebo-treated counterparts (7).

Role of noninvasive testing. The primary role served by noninvasive measures of cardiac function is to define the patient population being studied and to establish that the cause of heart failure is systolic dysfunction. Repeat measurements of these noninvasive measures during the course of double-blind therapy would seem to be of little value.

Summary

A variety of primary and secondary endpoints can and should be evaluated in the design of pivotal trials for a new drug for the treatment of heart failure. Yet, the success of the clinical trial program will depend on the consistency of the data rather the specific P values reached in a single study. Success in the approval process is enhanced by (1) a consistent logic underlying the use of the drug; (2) a large number of endpoints that support its efficacy; (3) a small number of the inconsistencies in the database; and (4) a paucity of concerns about safety.

REFERENCES

1. Pinsky DJ, Ahern D, Wilson PG, Kukin ML, Packer M. How many exercise tests are needed to minimize the placebo effect during repeated exercise in patients with chronic heart failure. Circulation 1989; [October 1989 AHA abstracts] (in press).

2. Packer M. How should we judge the efficacy of drug therapy in patients with chronic congestive heart failure? The insights of six blind men. J Am Coll Cardiol 1987; 9: 433-438.

3. Packer M, Medina N, Yushak M. Hemodynamic changes mimicking a vasodilator drug response in the absence of drug therapy after right heart catheterization in patients with chronic heart failure. Circulation 1985; 71: 761-766.

4. Franciosa JA, Dunkman WB, Leddy CL. Hemodynamic effects of vasodilators and long-term response in heart failure. J Am Coll Cardiol 1984; 3: 1521-1530.

5. Massie BM, Kramer BL, Topic N. Lack of relationship between short-term hemodynamic effects of captopril and subsequent clinical responses. Circulation 1984; 69: 1135-1141.

6. Franciosa JA, Park M, Levine TB. Lack of correlation between exercise capacity and indexes of resting left ventricular performance in heart failure. Am J Cardiol 1981; 47: 33-39.

7. Franciosa JA, Jordan RA, Wilen MM, Leddy CL. Minoxidil in patients with chronic left heart failure: contrasting hemodynamic and clinical effects in a controlled trial. Circulation 1984; 70: 63-68.

PANEL ON SURROGATE ENDPOINTS: CONGESTIVE HEART FAILURE AGENTS

Dr. Morganroth: Which of the surrogate end points can lead to an indication for a drug's use in heart failure.

Dr. Packer: I think in general one would like to measure as many things and see as many things go in the right direction as possible to build a package that creates a high degree of confidence a drug is effective in the treatment of heart failure. Not all end points are equal and I think that hemodynamic data provide one with certain kinds of assurances that one has an effective dose, that the dose produces an effect that persists and that it is of a nature that might be associated with clinical benefit. In general, that is an increase in cardiac output or a drop in wedge pressure and I am not certain that we have enough data to really discern which one is more important although there are individuals who think the drop in wedge pressure is more important than the increase in cardiac output. I think that when one has to dose, then one needs control trials to show that that dose actually does something which is clinically effective and by that, one would then show that the drug actually reduces symptoms using some measure of symptoms and enhanced exercise tolerance using some measure of exercise tolerance. One can be very creative as to how one measures symptoms in exercise tolerance in people with heart failure. The standards now in the field are not necessarily the most perfect instruments and I think there are lots of ways of looking at a variety of ways of measuring those two end points that will create clinical benefit. Both of those measures, that is symptoms and exercise tolerance, need to be combined conceptually with the concept of morbidity in heart failure. If you can show that a drug reduces worsening heart failure or hospitalizations for heart failure in a blinded fashion, those are very important end points that demonstrate efficacy. So all of those are related to the concept of clinical status: symptoms, exercise tolerance, and morbidity.

Dr. Morganroth: Most drugs may not be perfect to show all of those endpoints. What is minimally acceptable to be comfortable that a drug should be approved for heart failure? How many of those features do you need?

Dr. Lipicky: There is no surrogate to measure all of those things and after one has measured all of those things, they have to stack up appropriately and make sense from the vantage point of the direction in which they go, and hopefully some of them will achieve statistical significance.

Dr. Borer: I think that there is a parallel here with the problem that we face in studying anti-anginal and anti-ischemic drugs when you try to deal with symptoms alone. It is very difficult to hang your hat on a subjective response to a subjective questionnaire. On the other hand, I would think that if one had several variables from part of a large series of variables that were studied showing that the drug was active in a way that might be reasonable to associate with a reduction in symptoms, with making people feel better and you have evidence from questionnaires (New York Heart Association functional class data as poor as they may be). that in fact people did feel better and you had something else, it didn't have to be exercise tolerance, it might be reduction in number of hospitalizations for intravenous therapy for worsening heart failure that that might be sufficient.

Dr. Pitt: I would like to echo some of these things. I think we would all agree certainly that survival would be acceptable. The difficulty becomes with some of these other end points. I personally would not be happy if quality of life was the only thing that was shown, but I certainly would accept two things, exercise and quality of life. It turns out that exercise is very difficult and in certain drugs it may not be a benefit yet there may be an overall benefit for the drug. I would argue that we ought to be looking at need for hospitalization as another end point and I think if we show quality of life and the incidence of hospitalization for manifest failure were less, I would think that would be a reasonable package. In the Dig-Captopril trial, we were able to show that both dig and Captopril reduced the instance of manifest heart failure as manifested by either emergency room visits or hospitalization compared to the group that was on diuretic alone. I think given the right kind of population, one would have an event rate which was reasonable, certainly less than the event rates needed for mortality I think if it went along with quality of life, I would accept that even if the exercise was zero.

Dr. Temple: I would like to know what you mean by quality of life. You mean the usual symptoms of heart failure disappear. I think people would be impressed with that. I would be worried about a more vague scale that perhaps was reflecting some CNS effect.

Dr. Pitt: I started off saying that I wouldn't accept the quality of life as the sole thing. I would if it was combined with the reduced need for hospitalization and one could show a significant in a blinded trial reduced hospitalization that would imply tremendous cost difference as well as the quality of life. Clearly we would want our patients to be home rather than in the hospital, aside from all the costs. Would you buy that?

Dr. Temple: Reduced hospitalization seems like a reasonable end point as long as the reason for hospitalization is reasonably well characterized and it makes sense. What I think Dr. Lipicky was saying is you would like to see the thing make a coherent picture. Not every end point needs to be significant at the conventional value. If some of them go this way, if you get reduced hospitalizations but symptoms aren't touched, you would have to wonder what is going on. I guess I think that exercise tolerance so far has proved not too bad a measure. Not everybody is lucky enough to hit on everything like the first Catopril trial, but when other trials have had difficulty, they haven't just had difficulty on exercise tolerance. They have had difficulty on other measures too, New York Heart Association and so on. So far it seems like a pretty good measure. I guess you can imagine drugs that wouldn't be expected to have much effect on that measure and if it didn't increase cardiac output at all, but somehow decreased wedge pressure, maybe you wouldn't expect much of an effect on exercise tolerance. I don't think anyone feels absolute about any one of them, and I guess I generally agree with what you are saying.

Dr. Pitt: One last comment. I think one of the next series of drugs that need to be looked at seriously in heart failure are the beta blockers and some of them may show improvements and some may not. That doesn't necessarily mean that they are not good drugs in heart failure. I think that is where we may have to re-look at some of this data.

Dr. Cohn: I think the problem is that we are dealing with a syndrome that has at least several different aspects to it and the agenda for management has variable endpoints. Certainly relief of symptoms is a primary goal in a patient who is suffering overt symptoms of heart failure. The quickest way to make a patient with overt congestive symptoms better and improve their exercise tolerance and allow them to lie down, is to give a diuretic and of course we use diuretics as background therapy and anybody who is congested can be improved by an increase in the diuretic dose. So from a symptom stand point there is no question you could demonstrate very neatly if you were willing to have a group of people with congestion on a placebo which of course you won't do anymore and a group on a diuretic that their symptoms would be relieved. That is certainly not the whole agenda in heart failure. We also have to worry about progression of the disease and premature mortality and that may be quite separate from symptom relief. It is entirely possible that one would find a therapy which when added to a diuretic and digoxin produced no further improvement in symptoms because the patient is basically fairly asymptomatic but would prolong his life by preventing progression of the disease. That would indeed be an appropriate therapy to add to existing therapy in heart failure because everything we are talking about is adding drugs to existing therapy. We are not talking about mono-therapy like we would with a drug to lower blood pressure. We are talking about background therapy because everybody with overt heart failure is on some form of background therapy already. Then you get into the issue of the quantitation of the symptom relief and in a patient population it is already being treated optimally with a diuretic and is therefore not overtly congested, you have to find somewhat more subtle quantitative end points for improvement in symptomatology. Most of the studies that Milton pointed out were really looking at peak exercise capacity because that is the easiest kind of exercise test to do. We all trained to do a progressive test to maximum. The fact of the matter is that it is a very poor replicate for what people do during their daily lives. Exercising to peak capacity is not something most of us do every day, but getting along at submaximal workloads in a more comfortable fashion is a common phenomena. You can demonstrate hemodynamically with some drugs that there is a hemodynamic benefit at submaximal but not at maximal exercise so one might not expect an improvement in peak exercise capacity but might expect an improvement at some submaximal load which is hard to measure. We haven't figured out a protocol to do this very well. We have to become more creative about trying to find a better way to quantitate improvement because I think it is a mistake to assume that if a drug doesn't improve peak exercise capacity the patient is not better. It is entirely possible to get better without an improvement of peak exercise capacity and then quality of life comes in and then we begin to wonder whether we can't find some surrogate for improved feeling of patients, their capacity to carry out their life activities, which we can't measure currently by any of our objective techniques. So it is a problem, but I think it is a mistake to think of this whole bushel basket and say heart failure is this one single syndrome and everybody is in the same basket.

Dr. Antonaccio: I think it is very important to remember that after consensus, the practical matter is in doing clinical trials with the new drug for congestive heart failure that you are on top of triple therapy already. It may very well be that an additional drug shouldn't be expected to produce all of the things that the previous triple therapy has already to its best degree done in these patients. You might expect, one, two, perhaps even a third type of improvement, but I think it is unfair to expect everything to improve on top of triple therapy. What is all the fuss about exercise capacity? To use the analogy that was made before with arrhythmias, you might get an increase in exercise capacity that demonstrates the drug does something, but so what if exercise capacity is not related to mortality. As far as I can tell, it is not related to functional capacity. It is not reproducible even with the same drug in different trials, the changes are very small, and it is probably related to changes in skeletal muscle blood flow than it is to any benefit on the myocardium, so why all the emphasis? I suspect it is because the drug that got approved, Catopril had that objective measurement increased and it is the one thing that they could look at and say objectively that this was a good thing, so everybody shoots for it. I really question in my own mind what the benefit is to the patient of some kind of increase in maximal exercise capacity.

Dr. Lipicky: I guess exercise tolerance has some significance at least within the context of the models that I bring to bear. It doesn't have predictive value with respect to mortality or necessarily known predictive value with respect to symptoms, but if the agent presumably is working in some fashion to make the pump able to pump better, the only way I know of being able to test the capacity of the pump is to in fact take it through more than just rest measurements. That is a necessary thing to look at it seems to me. The exercise part as far as I am concerned at any rate, and within the context of the model that I am thinking about is simply a means of being able to explore whether the pump is able to function in the body better. Indeed, the symptomatology associated with congestive heart failure and the ability to exercise longer may in fact be able to be brought together somehow and that may be part of the creative things where the evaluation of the data would not depend solely upon the ability to exercise longer whatever exercise tolerance end point one chose to use, but would depend on that and improvement of symptoms that one was able to devise a means of measuring the improvement of symptoms and thereby make it a combined thing. If a therapy somehow or another didn't seem to depend on a suitable alteration of the pump which may be a reduction of after-load or pre-load or it doesn't have to be an inotropic intervention as far as I am concerned. Then I think I would become less concerned with the exercise evaluatory part. I am comfortable with diuretics being there to relieve edema because one can measure that, would dearly love diuretics to measure other capacities of the heart with respect to exercise for example and to include that, but am comfortable since it has a specific reason to be used, that is to relieve edema. If something is "good for the heart" and is going to make congestive heart failure better, it ought to have the properties that it does that. In that sense, exercise has to have some value and has to have some weight and I would be reticent to think in terms of the therapy of congestive heart failure where exercise was not an important component of my coming to the conclusion that it worked.

Dr. Packer: I think there is a lot of potential for creative things. One thing we will see a lot more of in the future are perhaps exercise protocols or designs that are non-maximal. It is certainly a possibility and I think there is nothing in either the proposed guidelines or any of the discussions that have taken place that emphasize maximal exercise capacity. The only reason that it has been used is that it is perceived that the end point is more easily discernible and as you can see from the data I showed, that is not necessarily true either. Perhaps everyone is saying the same thing. If you measure a lot of things which are clinically relevant, either symptoms, number of hospitalizations, differential drop out rates for worsening heart failure, exercise capacity, either sub-maximal or maximal and the more that each of them go in the right direction is part of the package. Even if an individual component doesn't make it less than .05 if one of those points, and it happens to be exercise tolerance is .06 but everything else, symptoms are getting better, the differential drop outs, whatever it may be, but the more points you have going in the right direction, as long as the trends are in the right direction, I think that that gives you confidence that you have an effective drug.

Dr. Lipicky: Yes, and hopefully something will be below .05.

Dr. Temple: And you have replicated all that, too.

Dr. Borer: A good deal of the mud in the water with regard to some of the studies that have been performed over the last decade in heart failure has been due to the fact that populations aren't really adequately characterized with regard to the degree of systolic and degree of diastolic mal-performance individually. I think over the last couple of years people have become much more aware of this, but nonetheless, I think it is very important to attempt it at least. I think it is important to begin to consider characterizing as well as possible the degree of diastolic dysfunction in a heart failure population that presumably is being studied primarily because we think there is some degree of systolic dysfunction that is going to be beneficially affected by a pharmacologic agent. It may be that a good deal of the apparent ineffectiveness of some agents, in some patients, in some trials, is due to the fact that these patients have a good deal of diastolic mal-performance contributing to their problem and while one might be able to improve systolic performance to some extent than that might be a good thing, yet you are not dealing with a basic problem. We have all seen a lot of studies in the literature where patients have ejection fractions varying from 15 up to 50 and the 50 is not the same person as the 15. I would suggest that that is something that we might consider a little bit, certainly diastolic performance is difficult to measure.

Dr. Rector: If we are going to advocate doing multiple measures for chronic efficacy in heart failure, exercise testing, questionnaires, re-hospitalization rates, New York Heart Association, all sorts of things, does a sponsor have to do all of these measures in both pivotal studies to be acceptable?

Dr. Lipicky: More or less.

Dr. Temple: You probably should do exercise testing in both and the other measurements are the usual descriptions of how the person is doing. It doesn't seem especially burdensome to ask for symptoms, count hospitalizations etc. Probably the answer is you should do exercising testing, unless this is a drug where exercising testing for some reason just seems irrelevant and irrational. I am not sure that there is such a thing well defined yet.

Dr. Rector: Let's say you did the first study where the exercise test did not come out significantly different but on a well developed patient questionnaire, the patient's perceive a lot of benefit relative to placebo, so you have one study, and instead of making the investment to go out and do another major trial with the exercise studies which I do think require a lot of effort and cost, could you then go on and just do it with the questionnaire end points and hospitalization rates and need for concurrent therapy and things like that and drop the exercise test out?

Dr. Temple: To me at this stage, all of the drugs that seem to be likely to be a factor or have been have had a favorable effect on exercise tolerance.

Dr. Morganroth: Dr. Antonaccio, is that true? All the drugs you have seen have a benefit on exercise tolerance.

Dr. Antonaccio: You define exercise capacity as being beneficial to the patient. I don't see a clear cut reason to make that kind of statement. I don't see that there is good evidence that that is true for that patient.

Dr. Temple: That is really a different question and I don't think anybody has addressed that yet, but I would like to. Some measure of your ability to exercise seems very clearly linked to many of the complaints that people with heart failure have. One of the things they say is "I can't walk this far anymore. I can't shave". I get too tired" so exercise tolerance doesn't seem obviously irrelevant to all those things even if you could imagine a case where some symptoms might be improved without improving exercise tolerance. We are prepared to see something that is different but so far, there doesn't seem any reason to dismiss it as one of the things that is being measured. To me the burden is very much on someone who thinks that you can have a drug that is effective for all those symptoms and it doesn't have any favorable effect on some measure of exercise to make that case. I would not drop it as a measure at this point.

Dr. Cohn: But the patient may say now I can walk better, I am able to do the things I couldn't do before, but you do a peak exercise study and there has been no improvement.

Dr. Temple: I didn't say peak.
Dr. Cohn: I know you didn't, but if that is what the drug company has done.
Dr. Temple: In the old days, people used to see how far they could walk. Maybe that is a better measure. I don't think we are wedded to any particular thing. That is a common European test in claudication maybe that is relevant here. That is exactly what people complain about when they have heart failure, that they can't walk far enough.
Dr. Rector: Would it be acceptable as a measure of exercise capacity to ask the patient "Can you walk better?"; "Can you do these physical activities in your daily life better?"; a questionnaire as opposed to exercise?
Dr. Temple: That is not a measure. That is a patient assessment form and it has its own validity but these things are measurable. Actually the ability to discover truth is easier on the whole in measured things. There are less variable probably than questionnaires so it doesn't seem a terribly practical thing.
Dr. Lipicky: A direct answer to your question would be if one did what you were saying the trial where exercise tolerance didn't turn out but symptom questioned your check list did and then planned another study that left exercise tolerance out and just dealt with symptom checklists, that would not result in an application that would be turned down when it hit the door. It would be evaluated. It would not be a refusal to file. So it is acceptable. The probabilities of that being favorably acted upon decrease in my mind significantly as a consequence of having made that decision and I would not advise it but it could be done and it might fly.
Dr. Antonaccio: That is curious to me because it assumes the basis for the drug not having an effect on exercise, that could be a perfectly logical, pharmacological reason for a drug not to have a basis.
Dr. Lipicky: There could be but the thinking process that said that exercise did not turn out in one, therefore we didn't do it in the other is totally not acceptable.
Dr. Packer: I think part of the crime that is sometimes committed is not that something doesn't turn out, but that it wasn't even looked at. I think that sometimes doesn't want to look at things, because one doesn't like what one might find, but that doesn't mean that one shouldn't look. Sometimes you are surprised and it works out but sometimes it is a little self-incriminating to say you didn't look, particularly if it is something which might be as pivotal as exercise tolerance, but on the other hand, if there are other clinically relevant endpoints as hospitalizations and degree of worsening heart failure and one even in exercise tolerance study always looks at differential drop outs between the two groups. There is always a sort of key point in any analysis.
Dr. Temple: As a matter of practicality, it is much more likely to lose if you ask me for the vagaries of clinical measurements in general are worse than more rigorously defined measures. I think for example, that the movement from angina rate to exercise tolerance has allowed smaller studies to succeed, has allowed patients who didn't have enough angina to measure properly to be included trials and has made it possible to get anti-anginal drugs

approved, but angina attack rate, I think always gave the same answer. Not in the same patient all the time, but it was a perfectly good measurement too.

Dr. Packer: There is one trial, I am thinking of specifically, it happens to be with digitalis. It is the digitalis arm of the Captopril-digoxin study, which did not show an improvement in exercise tolerance but showed a significant reduction in worsening heart failure, rate of hospitalizations and emergency room visits with digitalis compared with placebo and there are lots of other studies that showed digitalis improves exercise tolerance. So this happens to be a particularly good example of a trial in which the primary measure of efficacy if one could use that was this sort of clinical deterioration rate which was more sensitive than the exercise tolerance.

Dr. Temple: You are bringing up a whole separate issue which is if you measure a lot of things you have a chance of winning on one of them.

Dr. Packer: Exercise tolerance went in the right direction, it just didn't reach $p<.05$.

Dr. Temple: I understand, but as part of this discussion that should be appreciated too. We're not just talking about being lucky on one, we are talking about a replicated observable finding and those measures are good measures.

Dr. Lipicky: Indeed, just talking about multiple comparisons, because if one accepts the stand being taken that you need a lot of things and they have to go in the right direction and some have to be statistically significant, you do get into multiple comparisons problems and in particular from the vantage point of design of clinical trials in congestive heart failure, our statisticians go crazy because they like to have the principle thing declared up front and all that sort of business and I discouraged that and they don't know how to handle it nor do I and indeed the multiple comparisons rules generally aren't applied here at least in the way we have been evaluating these trials which may or may not be a mistake, but it is the reason why I think that something has to reach the statistical significance but that everything has to make sense, the whole data base has to hang.

Dr. Pitt: If we use the example if I had a new beta blocker let's say that I thought would benefit from some clues that improved heart size, whatsoever and I a priori said "Look, my prime goal in this therapy is to reduce hospitalization and improve patient well being, and my goal is not to improve exercise." I think that that was stated a priori and when showed it in a statistically significant way, in a blinded trial and then could replicate that in a second pivotal trial, I think you have an approvable drug.

Dr. Morganroth: Do you? Without exercise tolerance data or success in exercise tolerance?

Dr. Temple: You might, you have certainly declared up front what your goal is and replicated it so you certainly don't have a multiple comparison problem there. You have identified the thing you want .

Dr. Lipicky: And clearly the goal there would be and it probably is from the vantage point of use of beta blockers of if one wants to have decreased one's ability to exercise because there is some other game and the protocols are oriented to along demonstrating what this other gain is and the degree to which exercise tolerance is even decreased in order to accomplish that goal, and it is a coherent story that fits, why not say sure that is fine? But the exercise tolerance business comes to me from someone says I am good for the heart and therefore I am going to make congestive heart failure better and I am being very glib about that, but then you have to have other kinds of data, but you can certainly have another position and say I have a useful therapy for congestive heart failure and that would indeed be a slightly different circumstance and it would require a slightly different data base.

Dr. Rector: As Dr. Packer pointed out, to date the efforts to measure symptoms by questionnaire or quality of life or whatever you want to call that have been quite varied and some of them have been more rigorous than others, in the FDA's point of view, what are adequate characteristics of a good "quality of life" or symptom measure in terms of what content should there be in those questionnaires? Do they need documented reliability within the studies that are being submitted to you and do you need supporting information that allows you to interpret these scores, these numbers, these measures adequately?

Dr. Temple: Personally I don't see any very good reason for resorting symptom scores at all beyond the usual measures that we use now. You asked the person, "How many blocks can you walk?, Do you have orthopnea? Do you have paroxysmal nocturnal dyspnea?" and then you see whether it improves. People have been doing this for decades. You don't need a sophisticated instrument. The question is whether you can show improvement on these things because they are relatively crude, but whether you gain something by wrapping all those symptoms into a score numbered 1-10 I think is very questionable and if somebody wanted to do that, then there is a validation process of checking out the success of such a score and characterizing people, but I don't understand the necessity for it. Why would one want to take the perfectly well understood symptoms of associated with congestive heart failure and blur them into something that comes out as a number and that nobody can understand. What is the benefit of that?

Dr. Rector: Here is a good example. A lot of people say are you more or less short of breath and the patient says yes, no. My point of content would be so what. What is the importance of that if we develop measures that measure not only patients' perceptions of how much they have shortness of breath or dyspnea has changed, but how important that is to them. I really worry about in the area of heart failure that we find something that is effective on an exercise time, but when we ask the patients has your life changed at all, they would say no, but if we asked them if they are more or less shorter of breath, they would say a little bit less, but it is not an important change.

Dr. Temple: You don't have to do that. You can ask them to rate it on visual analog scales. You can link the shortness of breath with the particular activities. You can be reasonably sophisticated about it to make yourself feel more comfortable with it, but I still don't think you gain by wrapping that plus four other completely separate things into some numerical score. Not that you can't do that and maybe would come to believe in it with time. One other thing, there are also well established activities of daily living type scores I don't know whether they are considered applicable to heart failure but they are certainly used in other settings. There is nothing wrong with that, it is just a little harder to pin down what you mean.

Dr. Rector: I think the main reason I would advocate having some type of patient aggregative scores is if we don't aggregate them, if we don't have the patient give us some Gestalt what the net benefit risk ratio is, then you are faced at the FDA and the clinician is faced with 20 different measures, some are showing improvements, some are showing worsening and you are faced with the physicians aggregating those and telling the patient, well overall you are going to get better on this drug and that may not be the same as asking the patient, if he has improved in one area, and worse in this area, overall, are you better or worse, and having the patient tell us, instead of some non-specific, non-explicit way if aggregating all those measures that you are taking anyway.

Dr. Temple: There are also well established uses of patient global scores, physician global scores. I guess I don't understand what problem this is intended to solve. It has been possible to consider approval of drugs for congestive heart failure, the ACE inhibitors are the best example, the problem with some of the other drugs is that they may or may not have favorable or adverse effects on survival, but the kinds of studies that look at exercise tolerance and symptoms seem to work out and give you the right answer. Why is this considered an important problem. It seems fairly easy to wend your way through the list of various symptoms and measurements so far.

Dr. Lipicky: I do think the thing that is missing from the kinds of things that are standardly collected are what impact that has on the patient's ability to live their every day life. Did it make the difference between not being able to work and being to work? Did it make a difference being able to shop for groceries and not being able to shop for groceries? Did it make a difference between being relatively independent and not being relatively independent of family and/or neighbors and/or relatives and therefore although we think we know that these patients got better, because they exercised longer, or had less shortness of breath or whatever, you really don't collect any information at all that allows any kind of value judgement to be made with respect to what meaning whatever it is those improvements were had to the patient and the patient's ability to just take part in everyday living. I don't think there is a standard test that people would agree to and I think one gets into semantic arguments when one says quality of life because they get sort of put into the context of some kind of numerical score that has some meaning, but there is no way of assessing whether any of the improvements that one thinks one has made in a patient's hemodynamics or exercise tolerance or whatever, what that meant to the patient and to the patient's ability to perform activities of daily living. That is missing totally from our valuatory data base.

Dr. Packer: Interestingly, we don't do that for any cardiovascular drug.

Dr. Lipicky: I understand that and I think it could belong. I am not sure of what the instrument should be and there certainly isn't any standard instrument that I know of, but it is a glaring thing that misses from every evaluatory part that we have.

Dr. Cohn: Let me go back to some issues about quantitative measurements. Peak oxygen consumption during exercise is a predictor of survival in congestive heart patients. There is a fair mortality over a fairly long period of time, more than a few weeks and now you begin to lose patients. You would guess that you are losing patients that have the lowest initial ejection fraction and the lowest initial peak oxygen consumption and if you are doing non-mortality on these patients, the placebo group or any group that has a higher mortality is going to naturally show more improvement than would the treated group in whom you are keeping people alive longer if the treatment is effective in prolonging life. That is an age old problem in terms of how you analyze the data. I am asking you, how would you advise people to do that. One way of course is to call the people who don't come back for a measurement because they are dead and give them a 0 which is obviously correct at that point and that tends to correct for the fact that death is an important end point and ought to be considered along with non-mortality efficacy end points, but that may distort the numbers a bit too. What would you recommend the best way to handle that?

Dr. Lipicky: I don't know that there is a way of handling that.

Dr. Cohn: The obvious thing is that if you find a drug which over a year has strikingly reduced mortality and you can't show any improvement of exercise, you might say, I'm not sure that drug is of any benefit, but you have kept all these people alive who would have had lower exercise and how do you justify the fact of the lack of exercise improvement may be related to the high mortality?

Dr. Lipicky: I guess you would lose the ability to actually use the exercise capacity as an end point and the material thing would be that in fact there was a differential drop out rate and that more people died.

Dr. Borer: If you have a drug that reduced mortality in patients with heart failure and didn't effect exercise tolerance or the Minnesota Quality of Life Scale or whatever, I think you would have an approvable drug for prolongation of life in patients with heart failure or whatever group of patients it is that you gave the drug to, which is a different issue than how do you deal with the drop outs due to mortality if you are looking at an exercise end point to show that people feel better on the drug which is a tremendous problem. I don't know how one would deal with it. Different statisticians have devised different methods and I don't know if there is a right and a wrong, although there is a right or wrong every time it comes up for approval with a given drug. One way however of dealing with the very important problem of non-comparability of the populations, that is the drug did well in keeping people alive who wouldn't have been kept alive, but the exercise tolerance was better in people in some other part of the group would of course be to either stratify for some variables that you think are important before randomizing or to attempt after the fact to show that the groups you were testing were comparable somehow which is what most sponsors do and seems not unreasonable. I think it is important to point out again the problem that Dr. Cohn raises here which is that survival and feeling better among patients with heart failure may not be due to the same things when you put people on drugs and you could have an approvable drug that makes people feel better as long as it doesn't make them die more frequently and you could also have a drug that makes people die less frequently without making them feel better. Although, none immediately comes to mind among the antiarrhythmic drugs, one might conceive of some wonder drug that somebody will invent next year that reduces mortality due to its membrane active effects in people with heart failure but it really doesn't do very much to exercise tolerance.

Dr. Pitt: I would like to challenge something Dr. Cohn said, where he said there is a good correlation between ejection fraction and peak oxygen consumption in survival. That is probably true in the drugs that we have looked at, the vasodilators, but it doesn't necessarily hold in other classes of drugs.

Dr. Cohn: I am talking about baseline, not therapy at all. I am just saying take a group of people baseline and measure their peak pO2, their peak pO2 correlates inversely with survival.

Dr. Pitt: But not the effect on drug?

Dr. Cohn: I think with vasodilators, ejection fraction increment in BHAT was a surrogate for survival, but we don't know if that would occur with any other drug. The change in exercise tolerance was not a surrogate for survival and that is further evidence that ejection fraction and exercise tolerance are rather independent measures of sickness but they both at baseline correlate with survival.

Dr. Packer: I think one way of grapple with the differential drop out issue that was talked about before, it is hard to use Dr. Cohn's suggestion and assign a zero value for someone who died because their major arrhythmic of death, an arrhythmic mechanism may or may not reflect the kind of symptomatology that you are trying to improve with heart failure.

Dr. Cohn: Because they are dead, they can't exercise. There may be exceptions to that rule.

Dr. Packer: I think it would be fair to look at rate of worsening heart failure which is clearly something related to the symptomatology of heart failure and rank that appropriately if that were going to do that kind of analysis into a modified exercise analysis. In other words, if an exercise protocol for instance reached a p value of .08 and one wanted desperately to get it down to a p value less than .05 and one found in looking at the analysis that much more people had worsening heart failure on placebo than on active drug, and one could factor in the worsening heart failure rate into a statistical analysis that would give one extra confidence that one was dealing with a real effect, in other words to use worsening heart failure as the worst possible and drop out because of worsening heart failure as the worst possible exercise tolerance in a rank type analysis or something.

Dr. Temple: Dr. Cohn was worried particularly about the possibility that keeping sicker people in the treatment group might make survival look worse in that group and the remedy for that I think is straight forward which is to follow the people who drop out and at least for mortality do an intent to treat analysis which if the problem he is worried about occurred, should make things come out all right because you will see lots of deaths in the sick patients who dropped out while they were on placebo and it will show that the drug wasn't doing it.

Dr. Cohn: That wasn't my concern, but if it were, you answered it.

14

TESTING THE RELATIONSHIP BETWEEN CHOLESTEROL LOWERING AND CARDIOVASCULAR DISEASE---PAST, PRESENT, AND PROSPECTS

Dr. Robert I. Levy and Dr. Conrad Blum

INTRODUCTION

The past 20 years has seen the completion of nearly 20 major clinical trials designed to determine whether treatment of hypercholesterolemia can prevent atherosclerotic vascular disease. The groundwork for these clinical trials was laid by a century of morphologic, biochemical, genetic, and epidemiologic experimentation showing that cholesterol plays a critical role in atherogenesis. Prospective epidemiological studies have shown the relationship between serum cholesterol concentration and risk of coronary heart disease (CHD) to be continuous and graded. Genetic studies of familial hypercholesterolemia have shown that affected men (with serum cholesterol levels 280-400 mg/dl) have more than a 50% likelihood of developing CHD by age 60. Furthermore, studies of atherosclerotic lesions show that the cholesterol in these lesions has its origin in plasma low density lipoprotein.

The evidence has fulfilled all of the criteria for the etiologic nature of an association: the association is strong and graded; hypercholesterolemia precedes the appearance of CHD; the association is independent of other known risk factors, and it is highly predictive when applied to new populations; it is consistent among different populations and in varied ethnic groups; finally, the epidemiological studies are in agreement with biochemical and tissue culture experimenters and with experiments involving intact animals (i.e., it is biologically plausible).

CONSIDERATIONS IN THE DESIGN OF CLINICAL TRIALS OF CHOLESTEROL LOWERING

The clinical trials of cholesterol lowering were designed to provide the final proof of the cholesterol-CHD connection. Many of the earlier trials, however, were compromised by faults in their design (inadequate sample size, inadequate control group, lack of adherence, randomization, or blinding) that led to inconclusive or unconvincing results. A statistically significant benefit with respect to the "hard" endpoints (definite myocardial infarction and CHD death) was not found in the earlier studies. The problem has been that until the early 1970s, the statistical issues involved in attempting to prove the lipid hypothesis were neither closely examined nor understood. Two important factors in any clinical trial are termed alpha and beta (Table 1). Alpha factors help to ensure that differences found are significant. Beta factors relate to the likelihood of detecting a positive result. The major problem with clinical trials of CHD reduction lies in the validated "hard" endpoints that can be measured today---myocardial infarction and CHD death. Even in a population with existing coronary disease, one can only expect a death rate of about 5% per year. Thus, any trial to demonstrate the effect of lowering cholesterol on prevention of CHD must involve a large patient population studied over a long period of time to generate an adequate number of events for differences to be evaluated statistically. Demonstration of any impact on all cause mortality is even more difficult because in any age range, unless patients with severe CHD are selected, CHD will normally account for less than 45% of the total mortality. Tomorrow, when (and if) noninvasive markers of atherosclerotic plaque progression can be accurately and precisely measured serially (MRI, ultrasound, computer assisted IV angiography) and validated as CAD endpoints, we may be able to greatly reduce the time and cost involved in clinical trials.

Other factors are also important in determining the optimal sample size for such a study. K is the fractional lowering of

Table 1. Factors involved in determining the power of clinical trials of the lipid hypothesis.

1. N: Number of subjects

2. alpha: Probability of positively interpreting a negative result

3. beta: probability of not detecting a positive result

4. Event rate in control subjects

5. K: Fractional lowering of risk in treated subjects

6. F: Delay to treatment effect

7. D: Dropout rate--loss to treatment

8. Duration of study

9. Adherence to treatment regimen

TABLE 1A CLINICAL TRIALS OF CHOLESTEROL LOWERING: SECONDARY PREVENTION TRIALS

Study	Sample Size	Intervention	Double Blind	Random-ized	Dur-ation (yrs)	Reduction chol. (%)	LDL (%)	Increase in HDL (%)	Endpoints (**primary**, other)	% red.
Coronary Drug Project (CDP)[1-3]	8341	placebo, niacin, d-thyroxine, or estrogen (high or low dose)	yes	yes	6	niacin:				
						9.9	n.a.	n.a.	7-yr follow-up	
									all deaths	1.6
									CHD death	3.1
									CHD death & nonfatal MI	13.9#
									nonfatal MI	27.3#
									angina pectoris	17.8
									15-yr follow-up	
									all deaths	11#
									CHD death	11.6#
						clofibrate:				
						6.5	n.a.	n.a.	7-yr follow-up	
									all deaths	2.4
									CHD death	10.4
									CHD death & nonfatal MI	7.2
									angina	(16.8)
									pulmonary embolism	(75)
Stockholm Ischemic Heart Disease Study[4]	550	clifibrate plus niacin vs. no treatment	no	yes	5	13	n.a.	n.a.	**all deaths**	26*
									CHD deaths	36#
									nonfatal MI	30

notes: n.a. = not available
( ) = increased event rate in treated group
* = $p < 0.05$
# = $p < 0.01$

TABLE 1B **CLINICAL TRIALS OF CHOLESTEROL LOWERING: COMBINED PRIMARY/SECONDARY PREVENTION TRIALS.**

Study	Sample Size	Intervention	Double Blind	Randomized	Duration (yrs)	Reduction chol. (%)	LDL (%)	Increase in HDL (%)	Endpoints (**primary**, other)	% red.
Finnish Mental Hospital Study[5-7]	5115[a] 5497[b]	diet	no	no	6	12-18	n.a.	n.a.	**CHD death, men** **CHD death, women** all deaths, men all deaths, women	53# 34 11 (6)
Los Angeles VA Study[8]	846	diet	yes	yes	8	13	n.a.	n.a.	**MI & sudden death** MI, CHD death, ischemic CVA, ruptured aneurysm, ischemic gangrene	20 31#
Minnesota Coronary Survey[9]	9057	diet	yes	yes	<4.5	14	n.a.	n.a.	**MI & sudden death**	(6)
Belgian Heart Disease Prevention Project[10]	19409	diet, anti-smoking advice, exercise, anti-hypertensive medication	no	yes	5-6	n.a.	n.a.	n.a.	**CHD death** **CHD death & nonfatal MI** **all deaths** nonfatal MI	20.8 24.5* 17.5* 26.1
UK Heart Disease Prevention Project[11]	18210	diet, anti-smoking advice, exercise, anti-hypertensive medication	no	yes	5-6	2.7	n.a.	n.a.	**CHD death** **CHD death & nonfatal MI** **all deaths**	8 (6) (11)

notes: a - first six years
b - second six years
n.a. = not available
( ) = increased event rate in treated group
* = $p < 0.05$
# = $p < 0.01$

TABLE 1C **CLINICAL TRIALS OF CHOLESTEROL LOWERING: PRIMARY PREVENTION TRIALS.**

Study	Sample Size	Intervention	Double Blind	Randomized	Duration (yrs)	Reduction chol. (%)	LDL (%)	Increase in HDL (%)	Endpoints (**primary**, other)	% red.
US MRFIT[12]	12866	diet, anti-smoking advice, exercise, anti-hypertensive medication	no	yes	7	2.6	3.4	1.5	**CHD death** all deaths	7.1 (1.9)
Oslo Diet & Smoking Intervention Study[13,14]	1232	diet & anti-smoking advice	no	yes	5	13	n.a.	n.a.	**CHD death & nonfatal MI** all deaths sudden death nonfatal MI	47* 32 74 55
WHO Clofibrate Trial[15-17]	15745	clofibrate vs. placebo	yes	yes	5.3	9	n.a.	n.a.	**CHD death** **nonfatal MI** **all major CHD**	11 26* 30*
LRC-CPPT[18,19]	3806	cholestyramine plus diet vs. placebo plus diet	yes	yes	7.3	8.5	12.5	3.6	**CHD death & nonfatal MI** all deaths positive ETT angina coronary bypass congestive heart failure	19* 7 25* 20* 21* 28
Helsinki Heart Study[20,21]	4081	gemfibrozil vs. placebo	yes	yes	5	10	11	11	**CHD death** **nonfatal MI** **CHD death & nonfatal MI** all deaths	17 37 34+ (6)

notes: n.a. = not available
( ) = increased event rate in treated group
* = $p < 0.05$
\+ = $p < 0.02$

TABLE 1D **CLINICAL TRIALS OF CHOLESTEROL LOWERING: ANGIOGRAPHIC TRIALS.**

Study	Sample Size	Intervention	Double Blind	Randomized	Duration (yrs)	Reduction chol. (%)	LDL (%)	Increase in HDL (%)	Endpoints (**primary**, other)	% red.
Leiden intervention trial[22]	53	diet	no	no	2	10	n.a.	n.a.	no comparative control group	
Helsinki angiographic trial[23]	28	diet plus clofibrate plus niacin	no	no	7	18	19	10	**coronary segments with lesion progression**	57#
									patients with lesion progression	75#
									CHD death	27#
NHLBI Type II Coronary Intervention Study[24,25]	116	cholestyramine plus diet vs. placebo plus diet	yes	yes	5	11	19	5	**CAD progression**	
									definite	54
									definite or probable	63+
									CAD regression	
									definite	34
									definite or probable	21
CLAS[26]	162	colestipol plus niacin vs. colestipol plus placebo	yes	yes	2	22	39	39	**subjects with native vessels with:**	
									new lesions	55*
									new closures	19
									subjects with grafted vessels with:	
									new lesions	40*
									new closures	50

notes: * = $p < 0.05$
+ = $p < 0.02$
# = $p < 0.01$

risk; this varies with the amount that the cholesterol level is lowered. In general, diet over time in a free-living population can only lower cholesterol by about 10-15%. With the use of diet and several drugs in combination, we can now lower cholesterol by as much as 50%. The use of medications alone or medications in combination, thus, holds potential for reducing the sample size and the duration of clinical trials of cholesterol lowering. With the success of the recent cholesterol-lowering trials, however, it is becoming increasingly more difficult to leave the control group untreated. The more aggressive and significant cholesterol lowering is in the control group, the more difficult it becomes to show the impact of further cholesterol lowering in a treatment group.

The F value relates to the rapidity with which a fall in cholesterol concentration leads to a reduction of CHD. For high blood pressure control as in the Hypertension Detection and Follow-up Program, the benefit of blood pressure lowering was immediately evident in year one. For discontinuation of cigarette smoking, risk decreases very rapidly in the first year and then more slowly. In two primary prevention trials of cholesterol lowering, the Lipid Research Clinics Coronary Primary Prevention Trial (LRC-CPPT) and Helsinki Heart Study (HHS), the time taken to achieve maximal treatment effect was 2-3 years. This delay is apparent in other studies as well, e.g., the nicotinic acid group in the Coronary Drug Project follow-up study.

The dropout rate (D) is a problem to be considered in any study. But in one that lasts for years a dropout rate of 5-15% per year can destroy an otherwise perfectly designed effort. Since a study with a longer duration will produce more events, a longer study has a better likelihood of achieving a positive result. However, increasing the duration also increases the number of dropouts, thus threatening the results.

THE CLINICAL TRIALS

Despite these problems of study design, clinical trials have shown that cholesterol lowering reduces CHD risk. Five major primary prevention trials, two major secondary prevention trials, and five combined primary/secondary trials have been brought to completion. In addition, there have been four positive studies employing coronary angiographic endpoints (Table 1).

The secondary prevention trials: Two major secondary prevention trials have been reported, the Coronary Drug Project and the Stockholm Ischemic Heart Disease Study.

The **Coronary Drug Project**[1,2,3] (CDP) was a large double-blind, placebo-controlled, multicenter trial of five different drug regimens (clofibrate 1.8 g/d, niacin 3 g/d, dextrothyroxine 6 mg/d, and two doses of conjugated estrogens [2.5 and 5 mg/d]) in the secondary prevention of coronary heart disease. Participants had a past history of myocardial infarction, but hypercholesterolemia was not a requirement of enrollment into the CDP. The mean follow-up period was 6 years. Treatment with high and low dose estrogens and with d-thyroxine was discontinued early because of toxicity. The clofibrate and nicotinic acid arms of the study were continued to the planned 1975 termination of the study. The clofibrate group sustained increased rates of development of angina pectoris, pulmonary embolism, and thrombophlebitis. In the clofibrate group, there was also an increase in gallbladder disease, increased appetite, and decreased libido. In the CDP, clofibrate did not cause a significant improvement in the primary endpoint (total mortality) or in other endpoints (nonfatal MI, CHD death, CHD death plus MI). However, cholesterol lowering over the study period was only a very modest 6.5%. Furthermore, data from the CDP placebo group suggest that the relationship between cholesterol and risk of future CHD events is somewhat attenuated after an acute myocardial infarction. In addition, CHD event rates in the CDP were less than had been anticipated when the study was planned. These factors could render inadequate the sample size for this trial. Furthermore, the lack of any lipid criterion for entry into the trial made the CDP less than ideal as a vehicle for testing the cholesterol hypothesis. Thus, the lack of a positive result for the CDP clofibrate group does not disprove the cholesterol-CHD hypothesis.

Treatment with niacin was much more beneficial. Although cholesterol was lowered by only 9.9% with niacin, the CDP was able to demonstrate a clear benefit from treatment with this agent. During the course of the CDP, niacin led to a significant 27.3% reduction in nonfatal myocardial infarction. At the planned termination of the study in 1975, there was a non-significant 1.6% improved mortality in the niacin group compared with placebo. However, when follow-up was extended to 15 years, a highly significant improvement in all-cause mortality became apparent at year 7 and was sustained through year 15 ($p = 0.0004$). Much of that improvement was due to reduced CHD mortality. The CDP was the first trial of pharmacologic reduction of cholesterol levels to demonstrate a convincing reduction in CHD.

The **Stockholm Ischemic Heart Disease Study**[4] was a 5-year, non-blinded randomized trial of treatment with nicotinic acid plus clofibrate in 550 male survivors of myocardial infarction. The non-blinded design of this study is an important weakness. Subjects were randomly allocated to treatment with the two agents or to no lipid-altering treatment. Cholesterol levels fell an average of 13% in the treated group, and this was associated with a 26% reduction in all-cause mortality ($p < 0.05$), a 36% reduction in CHD mortality ($p < 0.01$), and non-significant 30% reduction in nonfatal myocardial infarction. However, the open nature of this trial, and absence of lipoprotein measurements leave many important questions unanswered.

<u>The combined primary/secondary prevention trials:</u> These studies enrolled subjects both with and without pre-existing CHD. Three used dietary modification to lower cholesterol levels (the

Finnish Mental Hospital Study, the Los Angeles Veterans Administration Study, and the Minnesota Coronary Survey), while two attempted to modify multiple risk factors (the Belgian Heart Disease Prevention Project and the UK Heart Disease Prevention Project).

The **Finnish Mental Hospital Study**[5,6,7] involved over 10,000 inmates at two mental hospitals. They were studied with a cross-over design. In one hospital, the usual diet was prepared; in the other, milk was replaced by an emulsion of soybean oil in skim milk, and butter and hard margarine were replaced by soft margarine. After six years, the hospitals switched diets. Serum cholesterol fell by 12-18 with the experimental diet. CHD mortality was higher among men during the regular diet periods than during the experimental diet periods (pooled results: 6.6 deaths per 1,000 person years with experimental diet, 14.1 with regular diet; $p < 0.0002$). In this study, interpretations are confounded because subjects entered and left each of the mental hospitals in the course of the study. Although there were two periods of 6 years in the study, the mean duration of follow-up per patient ranged from only 1.36 years to 3.80 years. Thus, the patient pools during the two periods of dietary treatment were not identical. Some patients were transferred from one hospital to the other. Additionally, the mean baseline cholesterol level among middle-aged men in the hospital before treatment with the cholesterol-lowering diet was 30 mg/dl below that during the second dietary period. Thus, the populations studied in the two dietary periods seem not to have been comparable. Finally, the study was unblinded to the physicians who determined the cause of death. These weaknesses have rendered the results of the Finnish Mental Hospitals Study not fully convincing.

For the **Los Angeles Veterans Administration Study**[8], 846 men living in a veterans' home were randomly allocated to treatment and control groups and were followed for 8 years. The two groups were fed a diet with the same total fat content (40% of calories), but the treatment diet contained 3 times the polyunsaturated fat and 40% less cholesterol than did the control diet. The study was double-blind. Adherence to the diets was notably poor--49% of the potential maximum in the treatment group and 56% in the control group. For the course of the study, the cholesterol level in the treatment group fell to 12.7% below that of the control group. Cancer mortality was increased in the treatment group. However, analysis of this and four other diet studies with similar cholesterol lowering has not confirmed an association of cholesterol-lowering diets with increased cancer risk. For the primary endpoint of this study (sudden death and definite myocardial infarction), there was a nonsignificant trend in favor of the treatment group (52 vs 65 events). When other atherosclerotic events (definite cerebral infarct, atherosclerotic gangrene requiring amputation, ruptured aneurysms) were included, there was a significant benefit of treatment (66 events vs 96 events, $p < 0.01$). However, the validity of retrospective analysis with combined endpoints is questionable. Thus, while the results of the Los Angeles Veterans Administration Study are suggestive, they did not provide definitive proof of the cholesterol hypothesis.

The **Minnesota Coronary Survey**[9] was a double-blind randomized study of the effects of diet. The subjects were inmates at six mental hospitals and one nursing home in Minnesota. Maximum follow-up was 4.5 years. While the two diets contained similar amounts of fat, the treatment diet contained less saturated fat (9.2% of calories vs. 18.3%), more polyunsaturated fat (14.7% vs 5.2%), and less cholesterol (166 mg/day vs 446 mg/day). The treatment caused a mean 13.8% reduction in cholesterol. No significant differences or trends were found with respect to the study's primary endpoints (myocardial infarction and sudden death). However, this study was handicapped by the following factors: (1) serum cholesterol levels were low at baseline (mean 207 mg/dl); (2) many of the subjects were domiciled and ate the study's diets for only a small portion of the 4.5 years of the study; (3) many subjects (1892) were over 65 years of age and might have been relatively refractory to the effects of treatment; (4) many subjects (2632) were under 35 years of age and would not be expected to contribute many CHD events.

The **Belgian Heart Disease Prevention Project**[10] and the **UK Heart Disease Prevention Project**[11] were the two largest centers in the WHO European Collaborative Trial in the Multifactorial Prevention of Coronary Heart Disease. These studies enrolled factory-working men aged 40-59. Randomization was by factory. The intervention comprised advice on a cholesterol-lowering diet, cessation of smoking, weight control, exercise, and treatment of hypertension. The interpretation of these studies is confounded by their unblinded nature, intervention on multiple risk factors, and marked center-to-center variation in modification of risk factors and CHD rates. In the UK center, estimated CHD risk (calculated from changes in risk factors) improved only 4%, plasma cholesterol fell only 2.7%, and changes in CHD were minimal. In the Belgian center, where risk factor changes were greater (estimated risk improved 16%; cholesterol reduction not reported), the intervention led to significant benefit in total mortality (17.5% reduction, $p < 0.05$) and in CHD incidence (CHD mortality plus nonfatal MI) (24.5% reduction, $p < 0.05$).

<u>The primary prevention trials:</u> Five major studies of CHD prevention by cholesterol lowering have involved subjects without symptomatic CHD at baseline.

The **US Multiple Risk Factor Intervention Trial**[12] (MRFIT) involved 12,866 high risk middle-aged men who were randomly assigned to a special intervention (SI) program or to usual medical care (UC) in their communities. The SI program involved dietary treatment of hypercholesterolemia, exercise, antihypertensive therapy, and counselling to help control weight and cease cigarette use. It was anticipated that men in the SI group would sustain a 10% reduction in serum cholesterol, while those in the UC group would not evidence any change in cholesterol. However, the cholesterol lowering in the SI group (6.6%) was less than expected, and there was a 3.4% reduction in serum cholesterol in the UC group. Consequently, during the course of the trial the two groups differed only slightly in their total and LDL cholesterol levels. Several factors contributed to the disappointing degree of cholesterol lowering: (1) cholesterol lowering was not a part of the intervention program for 1/3 of the participants who were normocholesterolemic at baseline, (2) the prescribed antihypertensive treatment raises total and LDL cholesterol levels, (3) the phenomenon of the health-conscious volunteer led to a greater than expected cholesterol lowering in the UC group, and (4) the study was performed when there was a strong secular trend to lower cholesterol levels in the population at large. Because the difference in cholesterol levels between the two groups was so small, the MRFIT could not test the cholesterol-CHD hypothesis. The intervention, which did not cause a substantial difference in cholesterol levels between the two groups, did not lead to any significant difference for the study population as a whole in the study's primary endpoint, CHD death. However, among hypercholesterolemic normotensive smokers, the intervention led to a 48.7% fall in CHD mortality. It is of note that a very similar result was found when a similar (normotensive, hypercholesterolemic, smoking) population was studied with diet and smoking intervention in the Oslo Heart Trial.

The **Oslo Heart Trial of Diet and Smoking Intervention**[13,14] was a 5-year study of 1232 normotensive men aged 40-49 years who were at high risk of CHD on the basis of hypercholesterolemia (290-380 mg/dl) and an elevated coronary risk score (based on serum cholesterol, blood pressure, and cigarette use). They were randomly allocated to intervention (diet and antismoking advice) and control groups. The intervention group sustained a fall in serum cholesterol to 13% below the level of the control group; cigarette smoking was 45% less in the intervention group. The intervention group demonstrated a 46% reduction in the primary endpoint (CHD death and nonfatal myocardial infarction). There were also significant reductions in the incidence of sudden death (74%) and nonfatal myocardial infarction (55%). Total mortality was reduced by 32%, but this did not achieve statistical significance after 5 years. Multivariate analysis attributed a majority (60%) of the benefit of the interventions to changes in cholesterol and no more than about 25% to reduced cigarette use. When follow-up was prolonged an additional 3.5 years after termination of the study, the intervention still produced a significant reduction in CHD; additionally, there was now evident a marginally significant 36% ($p = 0.055$) reduction in all cause mortality.

The **Who Clofibrate Trial**[15,16,17] involved 10,627 men aged 30-59 years with serum cholesterol levels among the highest third of the population distribution. They were randomized to treatment with clofibrate or placebo. In addition, there was a low cholesterol control group. Cholesterol fell an average of 9% in the clofibrate-treated group relative to the high-cholesterol control group. This fall in cholesterol was associated with a significant 20% reduction in CHD and a 26% reduction in nonfatal myocardial infarction ($p < 0.05$). Subjects with the greatest cholesterol-lowering sustained the best reduction in CHD risk. In the WHO Clofibrate Trial, there was no significant difference between the groups in mortality from CHD; total and noncardiovascular mortality were significantly higher in the clofibrate group. A variety of diseases contributed to the increased mortality. There were non-significant increases in deaths due to cancer and several other conditions. The increased mortality was not related to changes in cholesterol. This study provides further evidence that cholesterol lowering can prevent CHD; however it suggests that cholesterol lowering by means of clofibrate may not be beneficial.

The **Lipid Research Clinics Coronary Primary Prevention Trial**[18,19] enrolled 3806 hypercholesterolemic men (cholesterol > 265 mg/dl, LDL cholesterol >190 mg/dl) aged 35-59 years for a randomized, double-blind trial of cholesterol lowering. The participants were randomly assigned to treatment with the bile acid sequestrant cholestyramine or placebo. Over the mean 7.3-year follow-up period, the cholestyramine group sustained an 8.5% reduction in total plasma cholesterol and a 12.5% reduction in LDL compared to the placebo group. This was associated with a 19% ($p < 0.05$) reduction in the incidence of the trial's primary endpoint definite CHD death and nonfatal myocardial infarction. Quantitatively similar reductions were found for other CHD endpoints: angina pectoris (20%), positive exercise stress test (25%), performance of coronary artery bypass surgery (21%). The two groups were identical in the number of malignancies to occur (57 in each) and were similar in the number of fatalities due to malignancy (16 in the cholestyramine group and 15 in the placebo group). There was a slight, non-significant reduction in all-cause mortality in the cholestyramine group (68 vs 71 cases). The LRC-CPPT had not been designed with a sample size large enough to expect a significant effect on all-cause mortality, so the lack of statistical significance here cannot be considered to be meaningful. Multivariate analysis showed that the substantial fall in LDL cholesterol and the small 3.6% increase in HDL cholesterol in the cholestyramine group independently improved CHD risk. Each 1 mg/dl increase in HDL cholesterol resulted in a 4.4% risk reduction. A linear relationship was found between the degree of cholesterol reduction and CHD risk reduction. Full compliance (24 g/day of cholestyramine) caused a 25% fall in plasma cholesterol and a 50% reduction in CHD risk. This study, thus, provided definitive evidence in man of the benefits of cholesterol (LDL) lowering.

The **Helsinki Heart Study**[20,21] utilized utilized the fibric acid medication gemfibrozil in a double-blind, randomized, placebo-controlled, primary prevention trial involving 4081 men with non-HDL cholesterol levels exceeding 200 mg/dl. While the two groups were similar at baseline, through the course of the trial, the gemfibrozil group evidenced a 10% reduction in total and LDL cholesterol and an 11% increase in HDL cholesterol. This was associated with a 34% reduction in the primary endpoint of CHD death and nonfatal myocardial infarction ($p < 0.02$). In both the

Helsinki Heart Study and the LRC-CPPT, no CHD benefit of treatment was seen in the first two years of study. Multivariate analysis showed the benefit of gemfibrozil to be mediated both by a reduction in LDL and an increase in HDL. The predominant effect appeared to be due to the elevation of HDL. Total mortality for the two groups was nearly identical. However, the number of subjects enrolled in the Helsinki Heart Study was too small for a significant effect on total or CHD mortality to be expected. Cancer mortality was identical in the two groups. There were non-significant reductions in mortality due to CHD and ischemic stroke; there were non-significant increases in mortality due to hemorrhagic stroke and to accidents and violence.

Angiographic studies: Four major cholesterol-lowering trials with angiographic endpoints have been reported. Two lacked randomized controls (the Leiden Intervention Trial and the Helsinki angiographic trial). The NHLBI Type II Coronary Intervention Study and the Cholesterol Lowering Atherosclerosis Study (CLAS) were carefully designed with randomized control groups.

The **Leiden Intervention Trial**[22] was an uncontrolled study of a vegetarian diet in 53 persons with stable angina pectoris and at least 50% stenosis of one or more coronary arteries. The subjects underwent coronary angiography at baseline and after two years. The diet contained 7% of calories as saturated fat, and 30 mg cholesterol/1000 Calories. Coronary lesion growth was found to correlate with the total/HDL cholesterol sustained during the two year duration of the trial ($r = 0.50$, $p = 0.001$). A major weakness in this trial was the absence of a control group.

The **Helsinki angiographic trial**[23] was a nonrandomized trial of diet, clofibrate, and nicotinic acid in 28 hyperlipidemic (cholesterol >278 mg/dl, triglyceride > 177 mg/dl) patients with coronary artery disease in two or three vessels. All subjects were instructed in a diet. If cholesterol remained over 232 mg/dl or triglyceride over 142 mg/dl, clofibrate (2 g/d) was added. If the subjects remained hyperlipidemic, nicotinic acid (1.5-2.5 g/d) was then added. Coronary angiography was done at baseline and after two and seven years of treatment. Twenty hyperlipidemic controls (nonrandomized) were taken from another prospective study being carried out at the same hospital. The two groups had similar cholesterol levels at baseline, but the treated group had a 30% higher triglyceride level. Baseline HDL cholesterol levels were not reported, and the lipoprotein levels in the control group during the trial were not reported. LDL cholesterol fell by 19% and HDL cholesterol rose by 10% in the treated group. Coronary lesions were found to progress significantly less in the treated patients than in controls. However, doubts are raised by the nonrandomized nature of this study.

The **NHLBI Type II Coronary Intervention Study**[24,25] was a double-blind, placebo-controlled study of 116 subjects with elevated LDL cholesterol (uppermost 10% of the population) and baseline coronary artery disease who underwent coronary angiography before and after five years of treatment with cholestyramine or placebo. The cholestyramine treatment resulted in a 21% reduction in LDL cholesterol (compared to placebo) and a 6% increase in HDL cholesterol. The cholestyramine treatment caused a significant reduction in the progression of coronary atherosclerosis.

The **Cholesterol Lowering Atherosclerosis Study**[26] utilized an angiographic endpoint in a two-year study of 162 mean who had undergone coronary artery bypass surgery and had baseline serum cholesterol levels 185-350 mg/dl. The subjects were randomly allocated to treatment with a low fat low cholesterol diet plus colestipol and niacin or with the same diet and placebos for these two agents. Coronary angiography was performed at baseline and at the end of the study. During the study, LDL cholesterol averaged 97 mg/dl and HDL cholesterol averaged 61 mg/dl in the treated group (160 mg/dl and 44 mg/dl in the control group). The treatment was associated with significantly reduced progression of coronary atherosclerosis ($p < 0.01$). Furthermore, regression of lesions was seen much more frequently (16.2% of subjects) in the treated group than in the control group (2.4%). Thus, the CLAS has shown that lowering elevated levels of LDL cholesterol can slow progression and may even foster regression of atherosclerotic lesions.

PROSPECTS

While the more recently reported clinical trials have provided convincing evidence of the cholesterol hypothesis (lowering LDL delays/prevents CAD progression), they have done so at great cost, and they have required years for completion. The Helsinki Heart Study had a price tag of over $25 million, and the LRC-CPPT cost more than $120 million. As indicated above, high cost and long duration are inherent problems for studies with endpoints of myocardial infarction and CHD death. Requirements for sample size and the related statistical considerations (alpha and beta, fractional reduction of event rate, delay to maximal treatment effect, and dropout rate) mandate a lengthy study with a large sample size when clinical CHD endpoints are used. Angiographic endpoints require a costly and invasive procedure that ethically cannot be introduced in primary prevention studies. Better endpoints might reduce the time for performing a clinical trial and might reduce cost.

On possibility is the exercise electrocardiogram. Because abnormal stress tests develop much more frequently than myocardial infarction or CHD death, requirements for sample size and study duration are improved when this endpoint is used. In the LRC-CPPT placebo group, a newly positive exercise test occurred twice as frequently as did the primary endpoint (MI or CHD death). Therefore, in that trial, the exercise electrocardiogram was the first endpoint to develop a positive result. In the LRC Trial, the development of an abnormal exercise electrocardiogram occurred 25% less frequently in the cholestyramine group than in the placebo group. The use of the exercise electrocardiogram as the primary endpoint for a study of cholesterol lowering, if acceptable to regulators and practicing physicians, could lead to obvious economies.

Another potential noninvasive endpoint for studies of cholesterol lowering is ultrasound examinations of carotid atherosclerotic lesions. This has the advantages of allowing serial imaging of lesions and of being relatively inexpensive. However, it does not provide direct evidence of disease of the coronary arteries. Thus, the relevance of carotid ultrasound measurements to coronary disease needs further validation. Furthermore, experience with this technique is recent and no positive or negative trials have yet been completed with this modality. Thus, additional validation is needed. Similarly, intravenous subtractive computerized coronary angiography, MRI, PET, and new more sophisticated ultrasound techniques, while holding much promise for the future are still in their technological infancy as far as the coronary circulation is concerned.

In summary, while we have overcome our initial innocence in approaching cholesterol lowering/CAD trials by improving study design, we are now at a crossroads. With the evidence in that cholesterol reduction reduces CAD morbidity and mortality and coronary artery plaque progression, we have a new dilemna. Ethical committees will no longer approve lack of a cholesterol lowering regimen for patient groups with high (and in many cases even borderline high) cholesterol levels. This will undoubtedly make future cholesterol lowering trials more difficult to perform and interpret. In addition, the long-term nature and high cost of trials that depend on CAD events (heart attack/heart death) as endpoints make such trials unlikely phase III or even phase IV studies by pharmaceutical companies in view of the shortened half life of drug patents. Thus, the next advances that will look at the benefit of treating even lower cholesterol levels or defining levels of cholesterol/LDL lowering/HDL elevation to produce atherosclerotic plaque regression will depend on the development and validation of better noninvasive CAD diagnostic techniques.

[1]The Coronary Drug Project Research Group. Clofibrate and niacin in coronary heart disease. J. Am. Med. Assoc. 231:360-381, 1975.

[2]The Coronary Drug Project Research Group. The Coronary Drug Project: Findings leading to further modifications of its protocol with respect to dextrothyroxine. J. Am. Med. Assoc. 220:996-1008, 1972.

[3]Canner, P.L., K.G. Berge, N.K. Wenger, J. Stamler, L. Friedman, R.J. Prineas, and W. Friedewald for the Coronary Drug Project Research Group. Fifteen year mortality in Coronary Drug Project patients: long-term benefit with niacin. Am. J. Cardiology 8:1245-1255, 1986.

[4]Carlson, L.A., and G. Rosenhamer. Reduction in mortality in the Stockholm Ischaemic Heart Disease Secondary Prevention Study by combined treatment with clofibrate and nicotinic acid. Acta Med. Scand. 223:405-418, 1988.

[5]Turpeinen, O., M. Miettinen, M.J. Karvonen, P. Roine, M. Pekkarinen, E.J. Lehtosuo, and A. Alivirta. Dietary prevention of coronary heart disease: long-term experiment. I. Observations on male subjects. Am. J. Clin. Nutr. 21:255-276, 1968.

[6]Turpeinen, O. Effect of cholesterol-lowering diet on mortality from coronary heart disease and other causes. Circulation 59:1-7, 1979.

[7]Miettinen, M., O. Turpeinen, M.J. Karvonen, R. Elosuo, and E. Paavilainen. Effect of cholesterol-lowering diet on mortality from coronary heart-disease and other causes. Lancet 2:835, 1972.

[8]Dayton, S., M.L. Pearce, S. Hashimoto, W.J. Dixon, and U. Tomiuasu. A controlled clinical trial of a diet high in unsaturated fat in preventing complications of atherosclerosis. Circulation 40:1-63, 1969.

[9]Frantz, I.D., Jr., E.A. Dawson, P.L. Ashman, L.C. Gatewood, G.E. Bartsch, K. Kuba, and E.R. Brewer. Test of the effect of lipid lowering by diet on cardiovascular risk: the Minnesota Coronary Survey. Arteriosclerosis 9:129-135, 1989.

[10]Kornitzer, M., G. DeBacker, M. Dramaex, F. Kettel, C. Thilly, M. Graffar, and K. Vuylsteek. Belgian Heart Disease Prevention Project: incidence and mortality results. Lancet 1:1066-1071, 1983.

[11]Rose, G., H.D. Tunstall, and R.F. Heller. UK Heart Disease Prevention Project: incidence and mortality results. Lancet 1:1062-1066, 1983.

[12]Multiple Risk Factor Intervention Trial Research Group. Multiple Risk Factor Intervention Trial: risk factor changes and mortality results. JAMA 248:1465-1477, 1982.

[13]Hjermann, I., K. Velve Byre, I. Holme, and P. Leren. Effect of diet and smoking intervention on the incidence of coronary heart disease: report from the Oslo Study Group of a randomized trial in healthy men. Lancet 2:1303-1310, 1981.

[14]Hjermann, I., I. Holme, and P. Leren. Oslo Study Diet and Anti-smoking Trial: results after 102 months. American J. Medicine 80(suppl. 2A):7-11, 1986.

[15]Committee of Principal Investigators. A cooperative trial in the prevention of ischemic heart disease using clofibrate. Br. Heart J. 40:1069-1118, 1978.

[16]Committee of Principal Investigators. WHO cooperative trial on primary prevention of ischaemic heart disease using clofibrate to lower serum cholesterol: mortality follow-up. Lancet: 2:349-385, 1980.

[17]Committee of Principal Investigators. WHO cooperative trial on primary prevention of ischemic heart disease with clofibrate to lower serum cholesterol: final mortality follow-up. Lancet 2:600-604, 1984.

[18]The Lipid Research Clinics Coronary Primary Prevention Trial Results: I. Reduction in incidence of coronary heart disease. JAMA 251:351-364, 1984.

[19]The Lipid Research Clinics Coronary Primary Prevention Trial Results: II. The relation of reduction in incidence of coronary heart disease to cholesterol lowering. JAMA 251:365-374, 1984.

[20]Frick, M.H., O. Elo, K. Haapa, O.P. Heinonen, P. Heinsalmi, P. Helo, J.K. Huttunen, P. Kaitaniemi, P. Koskinen, V. Manninen, H. Maenpaa, J. Malkonen, M. Manttari, S. Norola, A. Pasternack, J. Pikkarainen, M. Romo, T. Sjoblom, and E.A. Nikkila. Helsinki Heart Study: primary-prevention trial with gemfibrozil in middle-aged men with dyslipidemia. N. Engl. J. Med. 317:1237-1245, 1987.

[21]Manninen, V., O. Elo, H. Frick, K. Haapa, O.P. Heinonen, P. Heinsalmi, P. Helo, J.K. Huttunen, P. Kaitaniemi, P. Koskinen, H. Maenpaa, M. Malkonen, M. Manttari, S. Norola, A. Pasternack, J. Pikkarainen, M. Romo, T. Sjoblom, and E.A. Nikkila. Lipid alterations and decline in the incidence of coronary heart disease in the Helsinki Heart Study. J. Am. Med. Assoc. 260:641-651, 1988.

[22]Arntzenius, A.C., D. Kromhout, J.D. Barth, J.H.C. Reiber, A.V.G. Bruschke, B. Buis, C.M. van Gent, N. Kempen-Boogd, S. Strikwerda, and E.A. van der Velde. Diet, lipoproteins, and progression of coronary atherosclerosis: The Leiden Intervention Trial. N. Engl. J. Med. 312:805-811, 1985.

[23]Nikkila, E.A., P. Viikinkoski, M. Valle, and M.H. Frick. Prevention of progression of coronary atherosclerosis by treatment of hyperlipidaemia: a seven year prospective angiographic study. Br. Med. J. 289:220-23, 1984.

[24]Brensike, J.F., R.I. Levy, S.F. Kelsey, E.R. Passamani, J.M. Richardson, I.K. Loh, N.J. Stone, R.J.R. Aldrich, J.W. Battaglini, D.J. Moriarty, M.R. Fisher, L. Friedman, W. Friedewald, K.M. Detre, and S.E. Epstein. Effects of therapy with cholestyramine on progression of coronary arteriosclerosis: results of the NHLBI Type II Coronary Intervention Study. Circulation 69:313-324, 1984.

[25]Levy, R.I., J.F. Brensike, S.E. Epstein, S.F. Kelsey, E.R. Passamani, J.M. Richardson, I.K. Loh, N.J. Stone, R.F. Aldrich, J.W. Battaglini, D.J. Moriarty, M.L. Fisher, L. Friedman, W. Friedewald, and K.M. Detre. the influence of changes in lipid values induced by cholestryamine and diet on progression of coronary artery disease: results of the NHLBI Type II Coronary Intervention Study. Circulation 69:325-337, 1984.

[26]Blankenhorn, D.H., S.A. Nessim, R.L. Johnson, M.E. Sanmarco, S.P. Azen, and L. Cashin-Hemphill. Beneficial effects of combined colestipol-niacin therapy on coronary atherosclerosis and coronary venous bypass grafts. J. Am. Med. Assoc. 257:3233-3240, 1987.

PANEL ON SURROGATE ENDPOINTS: HYPOLIPIDEMIC AGENTS

Dr. Morganroth: How comfortable are you with the ability to extrapolate from LDL lowering as a surrogate endpoint for the reduction in heart attacks for approval of a new agent? Is that sufficient for approvability in order to estimate risk benefit or are you concerned about requiring more than just simple biochemical reduction of LDL levels?

Dr. Pierce: I think to a large extent we've braced the LDL portion of the lipid hypothesis at the agency. However, I think we really look at each drug on a case by case basis. I think it is important to recognize that when the policy was formulated years ago to approve agents to lower total LDL cholesterol on that basis using that modification of risk factor rather than requiring a demonstrated benefit to the patient in terms of lowering risk of clinical events that the levels of cholesterol and LDL cholesterol that were being treated with drug in patients were higher than are presently recommended with the National Cholesterol Education Program and that there is a spectrum of feeling on the part of clinicians about who is appropriately treated with drug in addition to dietary therapy and as we move into lower and lower strata of LDL cholesterol and entertaining drug therapy for patients I think it becomes more and more important for us to have security and the precision in which we are estimating benefit and risk.

Dr. Morganroth: Does that mean that if you were approving a new drug today that had it's principal action on lowering LDL that you would in labeling define for physicians while cholesterol level groups should be treated, or do you ignore those issues and just say indicated for the treatment of high levels of LDL after diet has been first tried?

Dr. Pierce: Historically we've done the latter. But if we had a situation where the pharmaceutical manufacturer had undertaken a study that was positive that demonstrated an effect on rate of progression of atherosclerosis or some vascular bed or a reduction in coronary event rates we would always emphasize in the labeling what were the characteristics of that population studied and we would point out that there maybe pitfalls in carrying the extrapolations of how you apply that data to other larger populations and how far you go with.

Dr. Morganroth: You have no data today in terms of having demonstrated arterial changes in specific populations on a particular drug. Have you had to had the experience of having to look at such data and write labeling on that in that regard?

Dr. Levy: There is the data that was presented at the end of the lipid clinic trial and the data that was presented at the end of the Helsinke Heart Study. I guess the package insert was changed in both cases.

Dr. Morganroth: Dr. Troendle, any comments on that in terms of your viewpoints on what needs to be shown in terms of LDL reduction without any other data regarding benefit to the patient as a approvability claim?

Dr. Troendle: I think we are pretty much committed at the present time to approving drugs that do change LDL favorably but at the time that this policy started we really weren't measuring LDL. We were only measuring cholesterol and triglycerides and I think we have come a long way and we are now measuring not only lipoproteins but I think that almost anything that comes along has to have some information, not from all of the patients studied but in some subgroup, on apoproteins. Now we would have to include the lipoproteins and all of the factors that have come up. But, it gets to the point of where our insecurity is about using just lipids is pushing us to measure more and more of these little things as we discover them because we don't want to approve something which is having an adverse effect on something else that we don't know about. I agree with the comments that Ross said we would look at the drugs on an individual basis.

Dr. Morganroth: Let's assume that an application came in which a drug showed a 50% lowering in LDL but total cholesterol was not much lowered and that the HDL was in fact lowered rather than raised. What would you require for approvability?

Dr. Troendle: That has not come up so it's not a resolved position, but I have the feeling that we would feel that it was impossible to evaluate the benefit without some information on some form of endpoint that reflected the atherosclerotic process. Now Bob was asking if we would accept exercise testing and I think that that is at least a step beyond the lipids that we have been accepting all along so it would certainly be helpful and it would be done on an individual basis and would reflect some of the othe things that were measured also. The experience with probucol has been one of the things that has driven our concern about approving drugs just on the basis of lipids. If we had known about its effect on the lipids we might of had a different effect.

Dr. Morganroth: The antioxidive mechanism is attractive from at least one view. Let's say, Dr. Slater, you had such a drug, what argument would you take with the agency to try to overcome Gloria's reservations about this confusion?

Dr. Slater: I think the example that Gloria cited about probucol is actually a very good one and that it bridges the gap of the question of antioxidive. The closer the the drugs mechanism of action is made known to imput directly into what we understand to be the pathogenesis the easier it is for us as the sponsosr to make specific requests of the FDA and I think the easier it is for them to understand the request and to understand the drug in the context of its effects.

Dr. Morganroth: How much concern does one give lack of an effect on total mortality so far in the lipid trials?

Dr. Levy: I neglected to point out using those same calculation that if you use mortality rather than coronary mortality or heart attack you really have a problem because it is nice when you have a group with congestive heart failure, a group with serious life-threatening arrhythmias you know that heart disease is going to be the primary factor effecting outcome. But in a specially primary prevention trials and even in seconary prevention trials you can only expect that 40 to 55 percent of your patients here are going to sustain a coronary event as a cause of death and primary prevention at any age range other causes will be responsible for 55 percent of the deaths. You don't expect cholesterol lowering to impact on those 55 percent which means to get a study that is statistically strong enough to show the difference you need somewhere between 3-1/2 and 8-1/2 times the number of patients and I already talked about the cost of the studies that were done so I don't feel uncomfortable. None of the studies that have been done or that I have done have beend designed to show an effect on mortality. That's really such a great challenge.

Dr. Morganroth: Let me ask you a question about the niacin trial. What percent of the patients were still on niacin after five years?

Dr. Levy: The vast majority of the patients only had their cholesterol lowered 9-1/2 percent for the first five years, less than 25 percent continued.

Dr. Morganroth: So that 75 percent were not on it so the question is was the better total mortality due to stopping the niacin or because of the effect of the niacin early on?

Dr. Levy: Well you had to have first started it for five years, so whatever it is taking this medicine for five years during the five years had a very statistically significantly impact on heart attack. There was a 27 percent reduction in heart attack compared to the placebo group. Whether it was that these patients had less heart disease burdeon and, therefore, over a long time showed up. The group is the Oslow heart trial which has been going on for about 10 years they are showing 0.51 significance in terms of mortality. And finally we have the large population study in the US depending on the age, decade band cholesterols have fallen by a mean of 4 to as much as 9 percent over the last 20 years and during this time we have seen a reduction in both coronary and mortality. Of course the question is more significant in terms of the FDA.

Dr. Ross: What we want to really do is impact the bulk of coronary disease that occurs in this country then we are talking about changing the outcome with people who have for the most part rather average lipid levels so the ability to even detect a reduction in coronary risk in that population is rather formidable so our ability to detect the sum total of the cost of therapy in doing that is rather difficult. There are so many different things which could all add up and impact adversely on quality of life and duration of life. Many of the available agents that we have there are a lot of questions with respect to long-term safety we some potential for human carciogenisty and we've got this two year lag in the abililty to detect a favorable effect on coronary events with lowering LDL cholesterol where we have to think that we have a much longer lag in detecting the effects on potential carciogenic effects with some of these compounds. We have in some cases adverse effects on biosaturation. We have nephrotoxicity and neurotoxicity in some cases. I think that given that it's been estimated that perhaps there may be 10 million or so people in the US who would be candidates for drug therapy for altering their lipids. If they spend about a thousand dollars a year over about half a lifetime or so that is a considerable expenditure and I think we should try and take the long view and try to be creative in thinking of how we can cost effective and as practical as possible to get at the question of how we are effecting the overall benefit and risk namely total mortality. I think it is important and there is presently a pilot study organized by Dr. Peto in the United Kingdom looking at the effect on total mortality in a very cost effective way and we also have some ongoing trials that are looking at coronary endpoints with a variety of designs with lipid altering drugs. I think that it's important wherever possible to try to fund extensions of those studies where unlike in the case of the coronary drug project where people went off of niacin for the most part after five years they can be encouraged to continue in the treatment groups even after the unblinding and to try to get periodic data on mortality outcomes at various times.

Dr. Temple: The use of coronary events is not an uncommon endpoint in other settings. The post-infarction aspirin trials were most persuasive when you look at total events. They are less persuasive when you look at either cardiac mortality or total mortality. In fact, it would be hard to identify any of the individual studies as persuasive on their own for that endpoint. For primary prevention, the physicians health study the main endpont turned out to be coronary events. The mortality was too low to be a reasonable endpoint. But the LRC trial never sought to be a mortality study it was always intended to be a coronary event trial. But there is no question that death is black or white compared to whether or not you have an infarction and as one of three people who went and looked at the cardiac events I can tell you that if you had any doubts about the blinding of that study you would be nervous indeed. There is a lot of subjectivity in the question whether a person had a MI or not.

The LRC study that came out borderline significant using a one tail test and I can assure you there is some uncertainty about the exact numbers of whether each person had a MI. That's the way it goes. The effect is not that big and we were quite confident in the end that the study was well blinded and the decisions, subjective though they may have been about who had a MI and who didn't, were properly blinded. It is a much more difficul endpoint to feel very comfortable about and great care needs to go into defining the events. We thought in retrospect that the definition of whether you had a heart attack or not that trial was over complicated and made life difficult. Part of the criteria of whether you had a MI or not depended on whether you had the right kind of chest pain and unfortunately the description of the chest pain was made by the intern or a clerk who is not part of the study and does not know how much you care about it, so it can be quite casual and that made for considerable difficulty. All that said, there are alot of things to worry about when you are not using an absolutely endpoint. But still it seems to be a perfectly valid endpoint and it's been used in areas outside of lipids so I'm not uncomfortable with it.

I have just one other comment about shorter term endpoints. The further you get away from the endpoint that you are really worried about the less you know about some of the other things that the drug might do that might bite you. If you get an answer in a year and show that there is some regression of some lesion you never do get to find out whether strokes increase in four years.

<u>Dr. Levy:</u> A host of studies, many of which are bad studies, have been brought up again in the last period of time. The problem with a lot of cost benefit studies is that they give no credit to anyone alive after age 65 because they are on social security and not working. The problem is with a lot of these studies in terms of days or weeks related to some extrapolations done at the group at Beth Israel. They used a factor that was not correct in extrapolating from Framingham. They looked at the cost of taking cholestyramine each day assuming everyone took this drug. But in a regular study you would not be charging the patient for the drug if the patient is not taking the drug. The cost issues and the number of days one extends life I think they are all weak. They are referred to because they appeared

in the publication but they really aren't solidly based.

One can only come back to the results like the coronary drug project. You have to assume if you reduce the number of heart attacks the quality of that patient's life is going to be better. I also assume they are going to live longer.

Dr. Antonaccio: As it was pointed out we are certainly measuring new factors that we find in these trials. One of which is LP(a) although we know in general that this is related to increased mortality. I don't think we know much more than that and yet we are asked to provide this information. Provided the information is not a problem but I am wondering what you do when you get it? It goes in the wrong direction. For example, let's say you have an inhibitor that works perfectly well on LDL and HDL just like everything else but there is a statistically significant increase in LP(a). Is that a labeling issue or does that mean you have to go back and prove some clinical benefit with that drug?

Dr. Pierce: Fortunately, we have some trials ongoing which are going to demonstrate what the clinical benefit is and those are already in place. In terms of the 10 percent change I think this could be a labeling issue. My view of labeling is that it should be potentially helpful for the clinician for making his own decision with respect to therapy along with the patient. But I fully agree with you we don't know what the significance is of engineering a change in either direction in LPA.

Dr. Troendle: I think that the agency policy over the years has not been that you have to be better than or even equal to another drug if you don't have an adverse profile as far as safety goes that we can approve drugs that are less effective than other drugs because there will be people who are intolerent to the first drug. There will be people who are not responding to the first drug, and there is probably a place for another drug even if it isn't quite as good.

Dr. Morganroth: That's an interesting policy, is that the same policy you use Dr. Lipicky?

Dr. Lipicky: It just has to be at placebo.

<u>Dr. Levy:</u> I know the answer and I think it would be good for this group to know. If someone shows benefit in the carotid ultrasound or the aorta or the femoral ultrasound what would you allow to be said in the package insert and what would you not allow to be said in the package insert?

<u>Dr. Pierce:</u> I think I differ from Bob Temple on this in one respect. I think that for example if a agent were shown to stop the progression of atherosclerosis in the carotid arteries dead in its tracks, I'm not particularly worried about showing regression, in fact, showing regression then raised some potential safety questions. Anyway if you had that situation I would personally like to see that information relayed in the clinical pharmacology section of the labeling and I'm not quite so worried about misuse of that information in drug advertising.

<u>Dr. Morganroth:</u> How about if the sponsor proposed it as an indication?

<u>Dr. Pierce:</u> I was happy to hear Bob indicate the importance of validation of surrogate endpoints. Unfortunately, right now we are not really setup. We are doing about three studies to look at the carotids by B-mode ultrasound and we are using an index of medial thickness at various points. We don't know how really to best described a patient in determining whether a patient is doing better or whether progression is being arrested in terms of a global score and we are not setup in terms of the size of these studies to be able to have enough morbid events to know how if we do slow down but not arrest a rate of progression by a certain amount and what that means. If it's true that you have to have 75 percent luminal narrowing before you really start to appreciably be at a increased risk for clinical events and you only select people who mostly have 50 percent narrowing and you stop that then what does that mean?

<u>Dr. Troendle:</u> When we go to label a drug in the indication section we might run into the two studies rule which effects somewhat what we are willing to say in the indication section.

<u>Dr. Morganroth:</u> When there is a morbid or mortal endpoint, however, often doesn't one study seems to carry the day.

<u>Dr. Troendle:</u> That would effect it and we would have to see if the endpoint were actually morbitity and mortality that would have an effect on how we labeled it.

<u>Dr. Morganroth:</u> I would like to discuss long-term safety particularly when one is dealing with agents that are going to be taken for life. What are your current requirements for the degree of long-term safety that you need for approvability? How many patients, how long and what kind of tolerances do you use?

<u>Dr. Troendle:</u> I wouldn't like to put it in the terms of number of patients and length of time. I would like to say that these drugs will be used in essentially health men for long periods of time and the potential benefit is relatively small for the individual patient. In the LRC trial they treated almost 2000 patients for 7 to 10 years and saw relatively a small difference in the numbers of people who had events. When you are dealing with that low level of efficacy it seems to me that what you really need is safety studies that rule out a counter balancing toxicity, and if we could somehow have studies that are large enough to detect toxicity that would be off-setting. That would be what we need and it has to be looked at in an individual sense or in the sense of what you are going to accomplish with the drug.

<u>Dr. Morganroth:</u> But that has not been you policy up to this time.

<u>Dr. Troendle:</u> One of the problems that I have with approving drugs on lipid levels is that we don't know the benefit to risk very well.

<u>Dr. Morganroth:</u> Is there a change in policy that might be occurring?

<u>Dr. Troendle:</u> No, I don't have the power to change it. I can propose some change. But no at the present time we are still approving it but when you are asking what safety we would need that is what we think in terms of and we don't really get that.

<u>Dr. Morganroth:</u> I guess I should have asked the question what will be the minimum that you will require for you to sign off on approvability for a new drug that does a very nice job with lowering LDL?

Dr. Troendle: We have a track record on that. It is more or less about like the studies that have been done in this area.

Dr. Pierce: In recent past, the size of the safety database in terms of patient years of exposure has been closer to an order of magnitude larger than what we see in the guidelines for approval of antihypertensive agents.

Dr. Morganroth: When you say order of magnitude that suggests ten times more, is that what you mean?

Dr. Pierce: Yes.

Dr. Morganroth: Hypertensive databases would have 300 to 500 patients for a year with a total of 2000 patients to 3000 patients in the NDA. So, you are saying that you need 5000 for 10 years?

Dr. Pierce: No, I was using a 200 to 300 figure that had been thrown out yesterday at one point. But in recent past it has been on the order of 1,200 to 2000 patients for a year or more some patients being treated for three years. There has been no indication that that is going to be cut down any time soon. Really, it could very little bit according to the particular potential toxicities that look like what we were dealing with. There might sometimes be necessary to pin something down a little bit better preapproval. Which would result in the extension of ongoing studies.

Dr. Levy: Another area that's been dicussed which specifically in the cholesterol area which is to require phase four studies to do the kinds of things that Gloria has talked about to demonstrate long-term safety considering that these drugs are going to be used for long periods of time. I can remember being approached if the NIH would take the money that would be require to be spent by the pharmaceutical companies and do the studies for the companies. What is the recent feelings about the phase four studies as being mandatory and used or required in the lipid lowering area?

Dr. Troendle: We still do require phase four studies on all of these because we never have a database that we feel is really adequate on the safety issue and sometimes on the effect on atherosclerosis at the time of approval.

Dr. Morganroth: Has the Cardiac Arrhythmia Suppression Trial results influenced your concern about safety?

Dr. Troendle: I've always had concern about the real toxicity of these drugs.

Dr. Pierce: I think some of us felt that it validated our concerns that may not be too far out in left field in terms of the importance of long-term safety assessment.

PARTICIPANTS: TENTH ANNUAL SYMPOSIUM ON NEW DRUGS

Gunnar Aberg, PhD
Director, Pharmacology
E.R. Squibb & Sons

Mohammed Akbar Akbary, MD
Hoechst AG
Germany

Freedolph D. Anderson, MD
Executive Dir., CR&D
PRI Raritan

Deborah Anzalone, MD
Asst. Dir., Cardio-Renal
ICI Americas, Inc.

Keiko Aogaichi
Director, Cardiovascular
Research
Knoll Pharmaceuticals

Lawrence Asarch
Associate Director
Hoffmann La-Roche

Charles W. Ash
Sr. Scientist, Statistics
R.W. Johnson Pharmaceuticals

Steven A. Aurecchia, MD
Division of Metabolic &
Endocrine Drug Products
FOOD & DRUG ADMINISTRATION

Robert Bergstrand, MD PhD
Medical Director
AB Hassle

Dr. Paul Blake
Dir., Cardio-Renal Drugs
ICI Pharmaceuticals

Sharon L. Bonney, MD
Assoc. Dir. Medical Res.
Miles Inc.

Jeffrey S. Borer, MD
Prof. of Cardiovascular
Medicine
Cornell University

Magnus Brojer
Senior Director
AB Hassle

Jeffrey A. Brown, MD
Medical Director
G.D. Searle & Company

Robert S. Brown
Cardio Data Systems
Haddonfield, N.J.

Howard W. Bruce, MD
Director, Transderman
Therapeutic Section
Ciba-Geigy Corporation

Dr. Larry R. Bush
Research Leader
Hoffmann-La Roche Inc.

Dr. William J. Cady
Sr. Clin. Res. Scientist
Marion Laboratories Inc.

David A. Calhoun, MD
The Hypertension Program
University of Alabama

Dr. Lori Cirangle
Assistant Medical Dir.
Schering-Plough Res.

Catherine K. Clark
Dir., U.S. Regulatory
Affairs
Smith Kline & French

Robert J. Cody, MD
Research Dir., Div.
of Cardiology
Ohio State University

Michael R. Cohen, PhD
Associate Director
Sandoz

Thomas J. Colatsky PhD
Dir., Clinical Pharm.
Wyeth-Ayerst Research

Dr. Robert Colucci
Sr. Med. Res. Assoc.
Schering-Plough Res.

Glenn G. Cousins
Cardio Data Systems
Haddonfield, N.J.

Daniel Croteau
Clinical Res. Assoc.
Nordic Labs Inc.

J. Richard Crout
VP, Med. & Scientific Affairs
Boehringer Mannheim

Ellen Leigh Curtin, MD
Asst. Dir. Cardio-Renal
ICI Pharmaceuticals

Richard O. Davis, MD, PhD
Therapeutic Area Director
Bristol Myers

Dr. Ray Dawkins
Director Clinical Res.
Parke-Davis Pharm.

Dr. Hans A. De Hann
Medical Director
The Boots Company (USA)

David Deitchman, PhD
Dir., CV Clinical Res.
Bristol Myers Pharm.

Ellen Dempsey
Mgr., Clinical Res.
Cardiovascular
Nordic Labs Inc.

Leonard G. Dennick, MD
Clinical Res. Director
E.R. Squibb & Sons, Inc.

Philip De Van, MD
Dir. Clin. Res. & Dev.
Wyeth-Ayerst Labs

Elizabeth DiCesare
Medical Res. Assoc.
Schering-Plough Res.

Federico Dies, MD,PhD
Sr. Clin. Res. Div.
Eli Lilly & Company

Robert K. Dix, PhD
Sr. Assoc. Director
Pfizer

Lucette Doessegger, MD
F. Hoffman La-Roche
Basel, Switzerland

Dennis J. Donohoe, MD
Assoc., Dir., Clin. Res.
R.W. Johnson Pharm.

Jeffrey W. Dubb, MD
Dir., Clinical Dev.
Smith Kline & French

Gary Dukart, MD
Deputy Director, Cardio.
American Cynamid

Craig Q. Earl, PhD
Assoc. Senior Invest.
Smith Kline Beecham

Charles A. Ellis Jr.,MD
Andover, Massachusetts

Stewart J. Ehrreich, PhD
Senior Technical Advisor
Biometric Research Inst.

Robert Evans, PhD
Sr. Scientific Res. Assoc.
Lorex Pharmaceuticals

George Falcone
Director, Med. Marketing
A&D Engineering

Nancy Feliciano, MD
Assoc. Dir., Cardio.
Ciba-Geigy Corporation

John L. Fischetti, MD
Group Dir., Clinical Dev.
Smith Kline & French

Mary B. Fisher, PhD
Clinical Res. Assoc.
Merck Sharp & Dohme Res.

Harry P. Flanagan, DO
Dir., Medical Affairs
Wallace Laboratories

Michele R. Flicker, MD
Dir., Medical Affairs
Marion Laboratories

Graham J. Frank, MD
VP, Clinical Dev.
Parke-Davis Pharm.

Fritz Frickel, PhD
VP Research & Dev.
Knoll Pharmaceuticals

Mary Jean Fusco, MD
Asst. Clin. Pharm. Dir.
E.R. Squibb & Sons, Inc.

Thomas Q. Garvey III, MD
Pres. Garvey Assoc. Inc.
Potomac, Maryland

Donald Gieseker, PhD
Asst. Dir., Clin. Res.
Sterling Res. Group

Robert Glazer, MD
Asst. Dir., Cardio. Res.
Ciba-Geigy Corporation

Dr. Allan I. Goldberg
Associate Director
Merck Sharp & Dohme

Leonard M. Gonasun, PhD
Dir., Medical Research
Sandoz Pharmaceuticals

Maryann Gordon, MD
Head, Cardio-Renal
Hoechst-Roussel Pharm.

Sue Kurg-Gourley
Senior Investigator
Smith Kline Beecham

Jeffrey Granett, MD,FACC
Dir., Clinical Invest.
Smith Kline & French

Steven Grossman, MD
Sr. Clin. Res. Scientist
Burroughs Wellcome

Juan Guerrero, MD
Director, Cardio. Div.
Glaxo, Inc.

Susan Hannah, RN
Hoffman-LaRoche, Inc.
Glaxo, Inc.

Lloyd Haskell
Assoc. Med. Director
E.R. Squibb & Sons, Inc.

Susan Hedden
Mgr. Prof. Services
Knoll Pharmaceuticals

Dr. Alan J. Higgins
Director, Cardio. Res.
Hoffmann-LaRoche Inc.

Martha N. Hill, RN,PhD
Associate Professor
Johns Hopkins University
School of Nursing

Elaine J. Hinsch
Clinical Research Coord.
Hoffmann-La Roche Inc.

Terry Holcslaw, PhD
Asst. Dir., Clin. Invest.
Smith Kline Beecham

Rosemary Hoy
Product Manager
Merck Sharp & Dohme

Nancy June Hutson, MD
Dir., Metabolic Diseases
& General Pharmacology
Pfizer Central Research

Charles R. Ingram, PhD
Group Supervisor
E.I. Dupont

David Jackson, MD
VP, Clin. Res. & Dev.
Janssen Res. Foundation

Bradley Jefferies, MD
Assoc. Dir., Cardio. Res.
Reid-Rowell

Dr. Jerry Johnson
Dir., Cardiovascular Res.
Syntex Pharmaceuticals

Philip Johnson
Assoc. Statistician
Boehringer Ingelheim

Martin M. Kaplan, MD
Dir., Clin. Invest.
Boehringer Ingelheim

Abraham Karkowsky, MD
Med. Officer/Cardio-Renal
FOOD & DRUG ADMINISTRATION

John C. Kern, MD
Asst. Dir., Cardio.
Ciba-Geigy Corporation

D. Jeffrey Keyser
Mgr. Product Approval
Marion Laboratories

Edward B. Kirsten, PhD
Dir. of Clinical Research
Knoll Pharmaceuticals

Daniel L. Kisner, MD
VP, Pharmaceutical Dev.
Abbott Laboratories

Reinhard Kobelt, MD
Bayer AG
West Germany

Dr. John L. LaMattina
Dir., Med. Chem. Dept.
Pfizer Inc.

Kim D. Lamon, MD, PhD
VP, Medical Affairs
Rorer Central Research

Jeffrey R. Latts, MD
VP of Clinical R&D
Wyeth-Ayerst

Robert J. Lee, PhD
Sr. Med. Dir., Cardio.
Dupont Pharmaceuticals

Udo F. Legler, MD
Goedecke AG
West Germany

Dr. David A. Leibowitz
Forest Hills, N.Y.

Michelle Lener, PhD
Sr. Clin. Res. Scientist
Glaxo, Inc.

Blance Levitt, PhD
Sr. Clin. Investigator
Smith Kline & French

Gary Littman, PhD
Asst. Dir., Clin. Biostat.
Wyeth-Ayerst

Robert A. Long, PhD
Sr. Clin. Res. Scientist
Burroughs Wellcome

Rudolph W. Lucek
Senior Manager
Hoffmann-LaRoche, Inc.

James H. Ludens
Sr. Res. Scientist
The Upjohn Company

Mary Ann Lukas, MD
Assoc. Dir. Clin. R&D
Smith Kline & French

E. Paul MacCarthy, MD
Med. Dir., Cardiovascular
Miles Inc.

Daniel J. MacNeil, MD
Dir., Cardiovascular Res.
Bristol-Myers Company

Masahiko Maekawa
Deputy General Manager
Tanabe-Marion Labs

Sara A. Mahler, MD
Group Dir. Cardiology
Dupont Pharmaceuticals

Peter R. Maroko, MD
Group Director
Smith Kline Beecham

Pran Marrott, MD
Director, Cardiovascular
Berlex Laboratories, Inc.

Katherine P. Matthews
Asst. Dir., Clin. Res.
Sandoz Research Inst.

William D. Matthews, PhD
Group Dir., Proj. Mgr.
Smith Kline & French

Kandace Matzek, RPH
Mgr., Clin. Invest.
Boehringer Ingelheim

Craig A. Metz
Project Manager
The Upjohn Company

Wolf D. Michaelis, MD
Sr. Dir., Clin. Res.
Rorer Central Research

Shawn McDonald, MD
Clinical Res. Assoc.
G.D. Searle & Company

Mary McMenamin
Project Manager
Smith Kline & French

Charles F. McNally, MD
Exec. Medical Director
Rhone-Poulenc Pharm.

Joseph J. McPhillips, PhD
Assoc. Dir., Clin. Res.
Boehringer Mannheim

Dr. A.T. Monaghan
Assistant Director
Pfizer Inc.

Robert Munies, PhD
Dir., Regulatory Affairs
Janssen Res. Foundation

Michael G. Muro
Cardio Data Systems
Haddonfield, N.J.

Dr. Pauly Nancy
Roussel UCLAF
Romainville France

Thomas J. Nester, PhD
Asst. Clin. Res. Dir.
Beecham Laboratories

Jim O'Shea
Product Manager
Stuart Pharmaceuticals

Jillian Pincus, MD
Dir., Cardiovascular Res.
Ciba-Geigy Corporation

Bert Plekkenpol
Project Manager
Reid Rowell

Robert C. Pordy, MD
Asst. Dir., Cardio.
Hoffmann-LaRoche Inc.

Jerome G. Porush, MD
Chief, Div. of Nephrology
Brookdale Hospital

Harvey Raphan, MD
Dir., Reproductive Drugs
G.D. Searle & Company

Robert F. Reder, MD
VP, Medical Affairs
Knoll Pharmaceuticals

Dr. Stots Reele
Sr. Dir., Clin. Res.
Hoffmann-La Roche

Ziegler Reiner, MD
Clinical Research
Bayer AG

Rosann Reinhart
Project Manager
Smith Kline & French

Richard L. Riley, PhD
Dir., Cardiovascular
Rorer Central Research

Theodore F. Ritzer, MD
Dir., Clinical Research
Wyeth-Ayerst

Robert E. Robinson, MD
Dir., Medical Services
Merrill Dow Research

Edmond Roland, MD
Dir., Cardiovascular
Rhone-Poulenc

Gilbert M. Rose, MD
Associate Director
Wyeth-Ayerst

Dr. Alberto Rosenberg
VP, Clinical Research
Carter-Wallace

Morton Rosenberg, MD
Regulatory Affairs
Merck Sharp & Dohme

Peter C. Rueegg, MD
Clinical Research
Sandoz, LTD

Alexander Scriabine, MD
Dir., Preclinical Pharm.
Miles Inc.

Eugene J. Segre, MD
Senior Advisor
Syntex Research

David G. Shand, MD,PhD
Executive Vice President
Janssen Research

Shelton G. Sheps
Div. of Hypertension
Mayo Clinic

Lynne Smith
Sales Representative
Clinical Data

Jonathan B. Solsky, MD
Associate Director
Hoffmann-La Roche Inc.

Robert Speer
Dir., Medical Marketing
A&D Engineering

Jean Spenard, PhD
Nordic Laboratories
Laval, Quebec, Canada

Christolph Staiger, MD
Clinical Research
Boehringer Mannheim

Steve G. Svokos, PhD
VP, Reg. & Techn. Affairs
Knoll Pharmaceuticals

Dr. M.J.B. Tansey
Dir., Cardiovascular Med.
Glaxo Group Res. Ltd.

Dr. Michael D. Taylor
Senior Manager
Parke-Davis Pharm.

Jack Toukatly
Sr. Clinical Invest.
Smith Kline & French Labs

Orysia Tresznewsky, MD
Assoc. Dir., Cardio-Renal
ICI Americas, Inc.

Pedro R. Urquilla, MD
Sr. Assoc. Director
Pfizer Central Research

Dr. Vanderdoes
Boehringer Mannheim
West Germany

Elaine S. Waller, PhD
Dir., Cardio. Research
Marion Laboratories

Penny Walsh
MRA Manager
Miles Inc.

Susan Whalen
Sr. Clinical Scientist
Smith Kline Beecham

Dr. Kenneth L. White
Sr. Prod. Appr. Liaison
Marion Laboratories

Hugh Wilson, PhD
Sr. Drug Eval. Scientist
Marion Laboratories

Dr. Walter Wolters
Scientific Director
Cardiology/Angiology
Boehringer Mannheim

Joyce Zimmerman EdD
Associate Director
Hoechst-Roussel Pharmaceuticals